Revised & Enlarged Edition

DIABETES CONTROL
In your Hands

Dr. A.K. Sethi
(M.B.B.S., F.C.C.P.)

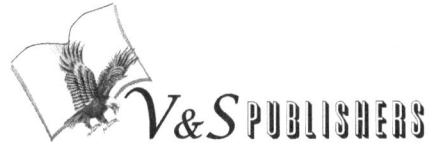

Published by:

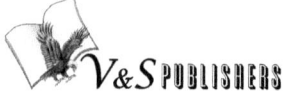

F-2/16, Ansari road, Daryaganj, New Delhi-110002
☎ 23240026, 23240027 • *Fax:* 011-23240028
Email: info@vspublishers.com • *Website:* www.vspublishers.com

Branch: Hyderabad
5-1-707/1, Brij Bhawan (Beside Central Bank of India Lane)
Bank Street, Koti Hyderabad - 500 095
☎ 040-24737290
E-mail: vspublishershyd@gmail.com

Distributors:

▶ **Pustak Mahal®**
   Bengaluru: ☎ 080-22234025
   Patna: ☎ 0612-3294193

▶ **PM Publications**
   Showroom: 10-B, Netaji Subhash Marg, Daryaganj, New Delhi-110002
   ☎ 23268292, 23268293, 23279900
   Shop: 6686, Khari Baoli, Delhi-110006
   ☎ 23944314, 23911979

▶ **Unicorn Books**
   Mumbai: ☎ 022-22010941

© Copyright: V&S PUBLISHERS
ISBN 978-93-813842-4-4
Edition: 2012

The Copyright of this book, as well as all matter contained herein (including illustrations) rests with the Publisher. No person shall copy the name of the book, its title design, matter and illustrations in any form and in any language, totally or partially or in any form. Anybody doing so shall face legal action and will be responsible for damages.

Printed at: Param Offseters, Okhla, New Delhi-110020

Preface

Diabetes is a dreaded disease which is known to mankind from time immemorial. In India there are about 35 million people who are suffering from diabetes. This accounts for about 25% of total diabetic patients in the world. Majority (90%) of these individuals suffer from type 2 diabetes which is usually detected accidently or in advanced stage. The World Health Organisation (WHO) has estimated that by the year 2025, the population of diabetic people in the world would reach 300 millions (presently 150 millions) and in India 57 millions. WHO has declared India as the Diabetes capital of the world.

Majority of Indian individuals suffer from the misconception that diabetes is due to excess intake of "Sweet Items" and will be "Cured" if they stop their intake. Moreover, diabetes is a disease which can be controlled but rarely cured by modern medicines. It has been observed that many diabetic patients improve dramatically when they combine Ayurveda, Naturopathy, Yoga, Magnetotherapy, Acupressure, Colour Therapy, Music Therapy and Feng-Shui with allopathic medicines.

In order to provide all this information for a layman, I have ventured to write this book and hope the readers will find it very useful and enjoyable to read.

Acknowledgement

At the outset I must thank Shri Ram Avtar Gupta, the Managing Director of Pustak Mahal who has given me the opportunity to write this book for laymen on an ailment which is widely prevalent around the globe. I am grateful to the patients who came to our clinic for treatment of Diabetes and benefited from the alternative forms of treatment provided to them. I am indebted to Shri R.L. Jaggi, retired Senior Accounts Officer (Northern Railways) who has been successfully practising in Chromotherapy and had provided me with abundant literature on different systems of Alternative Medicine. (Dr.) Swami Ananta Bharati, Chairman and Founder of Swami Keshwananda Yoga Institute has thoroughly guided me and taught me the art of Yoga, Pranayama and Meditation. Shri N.S. Dabas, an eminent astrologer and Vastu Shastri who is a staunch believer, follower and practitioner of Magnetotherapy has also assisted me in these fields. Dr. Ruma Banerjee, a practising physiotherapist and Naturopath has guided me in her field of practice.

My wife Dr. Sunanda Sethi, an Ayurvedacharya and a Traditional Reiki Master has been a source of inspiration. I thank my children Rupal and Mitali without whose cooperation this book would not have been completed.

—Dr. A.K. Sethi

Contents

Preface 3
Acknowledgement 4

1. What is Diabetes? 9-14
Structure and Function of Pancreas 9
Basic Cause of Diabetes 10
Ayurvedic Concept of Diabetes 10

2. Types of Diabetes 15-18
Insulin Dependent Diabetes or Type 1 Diabetes 15
Non-Insulin Dependent Diabetes or Type 2 Diabetes 15
Diabetes due to Diseases of the Pancreas 16
Diabetes due to Malnutrition 17
Diabetes due to Other Hormones 17
Diabetes due to Medicines and Toxic Chemicals 17
Diabetes due to Liver Diseases 18
Diabetes in Pregnancy 18
Types of Diabetes According to Ayurveda 18

3. What Causes Diabetes? 19-23
Age 19
Sex 19
Diet and Nutrition 19
Lifestyle 20
Infections 20
Medicines and Toxic Substances 20
Stress Factors 21

    Inheritance 21
    Causes of Diabetes According to Ayurveda 21

4. **Signs and Symptoms of Diabetes 24-25**

5. **Complications of Diabetes 26-39**
    Why Diabetes is Considered a Dreaded Disease 26
    When do Complications of Diabetes Occur 27
    Hypoglycemia or Low Blood Sugar 27
    Features of Low-Blood Sugar 28
    Ketoacidosis 30
    Diabetes and Heart Disease 33
    Diabetes and Kidney Disorders 33
    Complications of the Eye in Diabetes 35
    Complications of the Nerves in Diabetes 36
    Infections 37
    Gangrene of Foot 38
    Digestive System Disorders 39

6. **Diagnosis of Diabetes 40-48**
    Criteria for Suspicion of Diabetes 40
    Urine Examination 40
    Blood Tests for Sugar (Glucose) Estimation 42
    Glucose Tolerance Test (G.T.T.) 44
    Dextrometer/Glucometer 45
    Glycosylated Haemoglobin 47

7. **Treatment of Diabetes 49-119**
    The Objectives of Treatment of Diabetes 49
    Treatment Protocol 50
    Changes in the Lifestyle 50
    Dietary Management 51
    The Features of a Diabetic Diet 52
    Menu for Diabetics 54
    Types of Diabetic Diet 54
    Role of Physical Exercise 61
    Benefits of Exercise 63

Types of Exercises 64
Frequency and Timing of Exercise 64
Role of Yoga...65
Yogasanas...66
Yogic Kriyas 72
Pranayama 75
Stages of Pranayama 75
Rules for Pranayama 76
Benefits of Pranayama 77
Pranayama Useful for Treatment of Diabetes 77
Meditation 82
Basic Procedure of Meditation 82
Auto-Suggestion and Resolution 85
Naturopathy or Nature Cure...86
Hydrotherapy...86
Mud Therapy 88
Massage..89
Medical Treatment (Allopathic)...91
Ayurvedic Treatment of Diabetes...99
Home Remedies for Treatment of Diabetes 106
Magnetotherapy.. 107
Acupressure and Reflexology 109
Colour Therapy 114
Music Therapy 116
Feng Shui 118

8. **What Does the Future Hold for Diabetes?........ 120-123**
Better Diagnostic Facilities... 120
Better Treatment Modalities... 121

9. **Answers to Your Queries................................... 124-131**

10. **Role of Commonly Available
Ayurvedic Medicines... 132-136**

■■■

1. What is Diabetes?

Diabetes or Diabetes Mellitus is a disease in which the patient passes increased quantity of urine. Diabetes is derived from two Greek Words "dia" which means "through" and "betes" which means, "to pass". "Mellitus" is another Greek word, which means "sweet". In this disease the patient passes large quantities of urine containing a sweet substance, namely glucose. It is either due to lack of production of a hormone called insulin in the pancreas or due to the inefficient action of insulin.

Structure and Function of Pancreas

Pancreas is an important structure found in the abdomen, which plays a major role in the causation of Diabetes Mellitus. Pancreas is a soft, flat gland, which is 15-20 cm long, 3-5 cm broad, 2-4 cm thick and 80-90 gm in weight. It is situated in the posterior part of abdominal cavity just behind the stomach. Pancreas consists of three parts—the head, the body and the tail.

The head is enclosed in a C-shaped concave structure, the duodenum that lies between the lower end of stomach and the upper end of small intestine. The tail ends in a firm

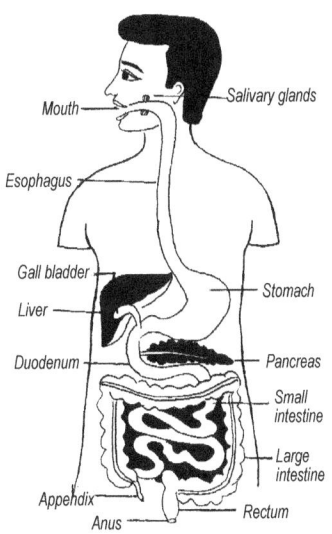

Fig. 1.1:
Pancreas & surrounding organs

organ, the spleen that is located in the left upper portion of abdominal cavity. The portion between the head and the tail is the body.

Functionally the pancreas consists of two parts:

The Digestive Part
About 99% of the pancreas consists of the digestive part. It comprises a large number of cells which produce the digestive enzymes which are important for the digestion of proteins, carbohydrates and fats in the food we eat.

The Hormonal Part
About 1-2% of the weight of the pancreas constitutes the hormonal part. A hormone is a chemical substance which is produced by an organ or a gland and sent to another part of the body through the blood where it increases the functional activity of that part. The hormonal part of the pancreas consists of large clusters of cells called the islets of Langerhans, named after the discoverer Paul Langerhan who discovered them in 1869. There are about two million islets in the pancreas. The islets consist of 4 types of cells:

- A or alpha cells produce the hormone glucagon.
- B or beta cells produce the hormone insulin.
- D or delta cells produce the hormone somatostatin.
- F cells produce pancreatic polypeptide.

Insulin is the most important hormone whose deficiency is responsible for producing the disease Diabetes Mellitus.

Basic Cause of Diabetes
Diabetes is mainly due to two causes:
1. Reduced production of Insulin.
2. Reduced efficacy/effectiveness of Insulin.

Ayurvedic Concept of Diabetes
In order to understand the Ayurvedic concept of Diabetes we must first understand the 3 bodily elements, which are responsible for sustaining the living body in their normal state.

These 3 elements are:

1. "Dosha"
2. "Dhatu"
3. "Mala"

Any imbalance in the 3 elements produces disease or ill health.

"Doshas" govern the physical and chemical functions of the body.

They are of 3 types:

1. "Vata"
2. "Pitta"
3. "Kapha"

1. "Vata" is responsible for active movements of different organs and parts of our body.

There are 5 types of Vata:

- **Prana** refers to functions of the brain and nervous system i.e. sensations of smell, taste, touch, hearing and vision, movements of upper and lower limbs, rectum and sex organs and breath.

- **Udana** refers to movements of the chest, diaphragm and voice box. It controls movements of breathing out, sneezing and speech.

- **Samana** refers to movements of the intestine along with digestion and absorption of food substances.

- **Apana** refers to the movements of the bladder, rectum, uterus and is important for passing urine, stools, menstrual fluids, semen and foetus (delivery).

- **Vyana** is concerned with movements of all kinds of both voluntary and involuntary muscles. It is responsible for movements of the heart e.g. blood vessels, lymph (special white fluid present in different parts of the body) glands and glands which produce hormones.

The diseases caused by the disorder of Vata are as follows:
- Asthma
- Epilepsy (fits) and other mental disorders
- Urticaria (a skin disease)
- Viral fever (due to temperature changes)
- Anaemia (lack of iron in blood)
- Obesity (Increased weight gain)
- Diabetes
- Diarrhoea or constipation
- Reduced functions of thyroid and adrenal glands

2. "Pitta" is responsible for the chemical reactions that take place in our body. It is of 5 types:

- **Pachaka** is due to digestive enzymes and other chemicals in the body, which control the digestion and absorption of food substances.
- **Ranjaka** is responsible for haemoglobin (the iron-containing pigment in blood) production.
- **Alochaka** is responsible for the biochemical activity of the eye, which is responsible for perception of vision.
- **Sadaka** is responsible for normal functions of the mind.
- **Brajaka** is responsible for removing waste products in the form of sweat and enhancing the natural glow of the skin.

The diseases caused by disorders of Pitta are as follows:
- Toxic fevers
- Hyperacidity (Gastritis)
- Vomiting
- Diarrhoea
- Jaundice
- Anaemia (due to destruction of bood cells)
- Bronchitis

- Skin diseases associated with pus formation
- All infections due to toxins, bacteria, viruses etc.

3. Kapha refers to promotion of growth brought about by secretions of different types of the body and organs. It is of 5 types:

- **Kledaka** refers to secretions of the mouth, stomach and intestines, which dissolve the food and destroy bacteria.
- **Avalambika** refers to secretions of the respiratory tract from the nose to the lungs and facilitates passing of air and flushes out foreign substances.
- **Bodhaka** is the watery secretion of the glands around the taste buds of the tongue which help in perceiving the taste.
- **Tarpaka** refers to the cerebrospinal fluid which is a secretion surrounding the brain and spinal cord. It provides nutrition to the brain and protects it from toxic substances.
- **Shleshaka** is the fluid lying in the bones and joint spaces called as synovial fluid producing movements of bones and joints with ease. The watery fluid surrounding and protecting the heart, and lungs are also referred to as Shleshaka Kapha.

The diseases caused by disorders of Kapha are as follows:

- Common cold.
- Infection of the lungs and other parts of respiratory system.
- Diarrhea due to infection.
- Jaundice.
- Eczema, pimples and other skin infections.
- Arthritis (painful joints).
- Rheumatic heart disease.
- Swelling and infection of the kidneys (glomerulonephritis).
- Peritonitis (swelling of abdominal cavity).
- Encephalitis, meningitis and other infections of the brain.
- Benign tumours of different parts of body.

Dhatu is a substance which is responsible for formation of basic structure of body. There are 7 types of dhatus i.e. lymph, blood, muscle tissue, fat tissue, bone-marrow, sperm or ovum.

Malas are waste products of various dhatus produced during the course of metabolic changes in the body. Examples of malas are sweat, urine, stool, gases, bile, ear-wax, nasal discharge, mucous secretions etc.

Thus disease is the imbalance of doshas, dhatus and malas.

Diabetes is one Type of disorder of the urinary tract in which patients pass excessive and turbid urine (PRAMEHAS).

There are 20 Types of Pramehas which are classified according to the doshas into 3 major types:

    Vataja Pramehas—which are 4 in number.
    Pittaja Pramehas—which are of 6 types.
    Kaphaja Pramehas—which are of 10 types.

Diabetes (Madhumeha) is a type of Vataja Prameha.

■■■

2. Types of Diabetes

Diabetes Mellitus is divided into different types, depending on the cause of disease and the situation in which it develops. Each type is distinctly different from the other by virtue of the cause of the disease, its presentation, complications, diagnosis and treatment. The different types of Diabetes Mellitus are discussed below.

Insulin Dependent Diabetes or Type 1 Diabetes

This type of diabetes is commonly known to occur during early childhood and adolescence. This is sometimes also known as Juvenile Diabetes due to this reason. It can also occur in middle aged and older individuals. In this disease, the pancreas produces very little or no insulin due to which the patient has to depend on artificial source of insulin. It develops suddenly and progresses rapidly. By the time it is diagnosed the patient may have developed many complications in the body. It is not commonly present in other family members. The individuals who develop this disease are usually not obese and have a normal dietary pattern and an active lifestyle. These individuals respond only to insulin injections and if not treated properly they develop complications and outcome may sometimes be fatal. The disease is more common in Europe and America. It affects 1 in 500 children and 1 in 200 adolescents.

Non-Insulin Dependent Diabetes or Type 2 Diabetes

This type of diabetes is seen in middle-aged adults and older individuals. This disease is more common than Type 1. It develops slowly and gradually and may not be noticed for years together. It is commonly detected when a person goes for a medical check-up before joining employment or before an operation. Such individuals are obese/overweight, voracious eaters and have a sedentary life-style. Often such people have other family members especially parents, grand parents, uncles, aunts or siblings with the same disease. The disease is not as serious as Type-1, with fewer complications developing and patients respond to oral medicines, diet restriction and exercise. The major differences between the two Types of diabetes are outlined below:

Differences Between Type 1 and 2 Diabetes

	Feature	Type 1 Diabetes	Type 2 Diabetes
1.	Age group	Commonly occurs during childhood and adolescence	Occurs in middle-aged and older individuals.
2.	How detected	Commonly detected only when complications have developed	Detected during official medical check up or before an operation
3.	Progress of disease	Develops suddenly and rapidly	Develops gradually and progresses slowly.
4.	How common	Less Common	More Common
5.	Body-weight	Usually normal	Increased
6.	Eating habits	Not contributory	Voracious eaters
7.	Lifestyle	Active or sedentary	Sedentary
8.	Family history	Family members not affected	Family members normally affected
9.	Treatment	Insulin injections are necessary	Normally controlled with oral medicine
10.	Complications	Develops early	Develops late

Diabetes due to Diseases of the Pancreas

Since the main cause of diabetes is the production of insulin in the pancreas, any disease affecting it will indirectly give rise to diabetes. The common disease/disorders of the pancreas are as follows:

a) Any infection of the pancreas
b) Tumour related to the pancreas
c) Any obstruction between pancreas and other organs due to stone, toxic chemicals etc.
d) Removal of pancreas by operation.

Such individuals may develop the disease at any age irrespective of their body weight, eating habits, life style and family history. They commonly require insulin injections for treatment while some may respond to oral medicines.

Diabetes due to Malnutrition

In developing countries like India many individuals in the adolescence and adulthood develop diabetes due to severe malnutrition. These people are commonly deprived of food in early life especially protein-rich food. Due to this they are undernourished and very lean and have very little production of insulin hormone.

Due to lack of food the insulin which is produced is also insensitive since it has no proper foodstuff to act on. Thus these individuals slowly devlop diabetes. They normally respond only to artificial sources of Insulin.

Diabetes due to Other Hormones

Some individuals develop diabetes due to excessive production of certain hormones which interfere with the normal action of insulin e.g. growth hormone, thyroid hormones, glucagon (from pancreas). Due to their interference, insulin fails to carry out its normal activities on the foodstuffs and patients develop high levels of blood sugar and hence diabetes. The features of such patients are variable and also their treatment.

Diabetes due to Medicines and Toxic Chemicals

Certain medicines and toxic food substances and rodenticides are capable of destroying the pancreatic cells, which produce insulin. This gives rise to diabetes.

Diabetes due to Liver Diseases

Certain infections, obstruction and other metabolic disorders related to liver also give rise to diabetes.

Diabetes in Pregnancy

Some pregnant women have been observed to develop diabetes during their pregnancy.

The different types of diabetes according to Ayurvedic system of medicine are given below:

Types of Diabetes According to Ayurveda

Diabetes is classified in two ways:

- Based on the Type of doshas. (Ref. Chapter 1)
- Based on inheritance. (heredity)

Based on Type of Doshas	Based on Inheritance
1. Vataja Type	1. Inherited
2. Kaphaja Type	2. Non-Inherited
3. Pittaja Type	a) Due to over-weight
	b) Due to under-weight

The Ayurvedic concept of diabetes is based on the imbalance of the 3 doshas, namely vata, pitta and kapha. When the vata dosha is predominant the type is called vataja and similarly pittaja and kaphaja types. Based on the inheritance theory the disease could be an inherited type in which there is diabetes in one of the blood-relatives, irrespective of the weight of the individual. In the non-inherited type we have 2 sub types: one which is seen in overweight individuals who are voracious eaters and have a sedentary lifestyle and the other subtype where the person is under-weight and malnourished due to lack of proper intake of food or chronic diseases like tuberculosis.

■■■

3. What Causes Diabetes?

Diabetes is a disease, which is due to multiple factors related to the individual and the environment and involves many systems of the body. Hence it is a multi-factorial and multi-system disease.

The various factors which contribute to the development of this disease are as follows:

Age

Although diabetes may occur at any age irrespective of the type, the majority of cases are seen in middle-aged and older individuals. Insulin Dependent (Type 1) and malnutrition-related diabetes occur in younger age group. In the latter group, the complications are more common, treatment difficult and outcome is sometimes fatal. Some researchers have also declared aging, as an important factor for diabetes and senile changes in the pancreas could also be contributory.

Sex

This disease is equally distributed in both sexes though in some countries, the male diabetics are more while in others, the females are more. The disparity could be due to lack of notification of this disease in hospitals since private practitioners treat many patients.

Diet and Nutrition

In obese individuals, Type 2 Diabetes was common due to resistance of body to normal insulin due to excess fat cells. People with malnutrition commonly have very little amount of insulin in the body and hence suffer from Type 1 or Insulin Dependent Diabetes Mellitus. Of late, research has shown that Diabetes may occur irrespective of nutritional status. Some studies have shown that children who are given cow's milk early in infancy may develop type 1 Diabetes. This is due to presence of "Bovine Serum Albumin"—a substance which may damage the insulin producing cells in the pancreas. Excessive carbohydrates, especially refined sugars may indirectly lead to type 2 Diabetes by giving rise to obesity.

Lifestyle

Lifestyle of individuals can prove to be a risk factor for development of diabetes in two ways:

Sedentary Lifestyle

People who have minimum physical activity or a sedentary life style are very much susceptible to develop Non-insulin Dependent Diabetes. The lack of exercise alters the action of insulin and its receptors.

Urbanized Lifestyle

Statistical evaluation of prevalence of diabetes in developed vs. developing countries and rural vs. urban population has shown interesting findings. People migrating from developing to developed or rural to urban areas show increase in the prevalent rate of diabetes.

Thus urbanized or westernized lifestyle promotes development of diabetes.

Infections

Infections both due to bacteria and viruses can precipitate diabetes in susceptible individuals. Infection of the pancreas can produce a series of events resulting in destruction of beta cells of pancreas, which produce insulin.

Medicines and Toxic Substances

Certain medicines e.g. steroid hormones and substances which increase the excretion of urine (diuretics) have been known to produce diabetes. Studies in animals using toxic substances e.g. Alloxan, Streptozotocin, Rat Poison (Valcor) have produced diabetes. Certain food substances e.g. Cassava and certain beans when taken in large amounts are capable of producing toxic effects on insulin producing cells due to high content of cyanide in them.

Alcohol when taken in large quantities over a prolonged period can prove to be toxic to the liver and pancreas and can promote obesity.

Stress Factors

Stress of any kind can precipitate diabetes in susceptible individuals. Stress may be in the form of surgery, infections, injury, pregnancy or mental tension due to different reasons.

Inheritance

The importance of inheritance in diabetes is seen in the following ways:

- Diabetes especially Type 1 is more commonly seen in the parents and blood relatives of diabetics than in general population.
- Certain markers - Human Leukocyte Antigen (HLA) when present in individuals signal the presence of diabetes especially Type 1.
- Many individuals with Diabetes especially Type 2 have other associated problems like obesity, hypertension and high blood levels of fat.
- Certain individuals have a defective mechanism by which the beta cells get destroyed by some self-destructive process.

Causes of Diabetes According to Ayurveda

According to the Doshas

Any imbalance in the amount of doshas in the body gives rise to diabetes. If the vata dosha is increased and the others are decreased, the type of diabetes is known as Vataja madhumeha.

Similarly in cases of increase in Pitta and Kapha doshas, the types are respectively Pittaja and Kaphaja.

Dietary Factors

Ayurveda has always implicated the cause of a particular disease due to ingestion of particular food substance. In the case of diabetes too, ayurvedacharyas have implicated increased intake of high carbohydrate and fat diet as the cause of diabetes.

People who have an increased intake of food substances like milk and its products, honey, sugar, wheat, rice, bajra, grains, meat, fish, eggs, ghee, oils, tea, coffee, aerated drinks and ice-cream are prone to develop diabetes.

Lifestyle

Sedentary lifestyle: People who are affluent doing more of mental work than physical e.g. politicians, shopkeepers, executives, zamindars, teachers, doctors and lawyers are very prone to develop diabetes. In contrast labourers, farmers, policemen, soldiers etc. carrying out more of physical activity are less prone to develop this disease.

Urbanized/westernized lifestyle: Due to the rapid urbanization and western influences, many people are ambitious, carrying on with irregular and high-caloric food and poor bowel and bladder movements and spending a luxurious life.

These people are highly prone to develop diabetes.

Lack of Exercise

Excess intake of carbohydrates and fat along with lack of exercise and laziness gives rise to increased body weight, which predisposes diabetes.

Nutritional Status

Malnutrition as well as obesity are risk factors for diabetes.

Psychological Factors

Mental stress, anxiety, depression and other psychological illnesses can also precipitate diabetes.

Heredity

Diabetes may be inherited from parents, grandparents and blood relatives.

Other Factors

Increased sexual activity, chronic diseases like tuberculosis (TB), piles, venereal diseases etc also give rise to diabetes.

4. Signs and Symptoms of Diabetes

The features (signs and symptoms) of diabetes are variable and depend on the following factors:

- Type of diabetes
- Stage of diabetes
- How it presents itself-abruptly or gradually
- Age of the patient
- Presence or absence of complications of the disease

Patients with uncomplicated diabetes may present to the doctor with one or more of the following complaints/symptoms:

- Passage of large volumes of urine, which is dilute and pale in colour.
- Passage of urine at night even in the absence of high fluid intake.
- Urine may contain "sugar" (glucose) which is not normally present in other individuals.
- Abnormally intense thirst, which leads to drinking of large quantities of water and fluids, irrespective of weather conditions.
- Sudden development of a voracious appetite.
- Complain of getting tired easily and a sensation of "weakness".

- In spite of increased appetite, loss of weight instead of weight gain.
- White marks on the clothes which are not easily washed off.
- Itching and redness around the genitals.
- Diminished vision with frequent changes of spectacles due to short sight.
- Slow healing of wounds as compared to normal people.
- Tingling (Pins and needles sensation) and numbness (diminished sensation) in hands and feet.
- Pain in the lower limbs especially the calf muscles which is not relieved by routine painkillers.
- Repeated infections of the skin, respiratory tract or urinary tract.
- Impotence.

5. Complications of Diabetes

Understanding the features of diabetes is incomplete without knowing the complications caused by the disease, how they present themselves and their treatment. Knowing the complications is important because Type 1 Diabetes always heralds its arrival along with complications. Type 2 Diabetes also gives rise to complications in the long run.

When a person is declared to have diabetes by his doctor the person receives a setback. He may think "why me of all the people? Many people enter into a depressive state with sadness and disturbance of sleep, appetite and concentration. Thus diabetes is a dreaded disease, a phobia and a curse for many.

Why Diabetes is Considered a Dreaded Disease
- It has very few premonitory symptoms before it is detected.
- It can only be controlled, never cured by modern medicines.
- If untreated or otherwise, it can lead to many complications.
- A diabetic feels socially insecure due to his dietary restrictions, regular meals and medications.
- A diabetic is not able to carry out stressful activities as compared to a non-diabetic.

The complications involve many systems and organs and occur due to various reasons. Their presentation varies according to the type of disease, the stage when detected, the organ involved and the extent of control of the blood sugar.

When do Complications of Diabetes Occur?

- When the person is suffering especially from Type 1 Diabetes.
- When treatment is not begun.
- When dosage of medicines/injections is less or more than required
- When treatment is not taken regularly.
- When patient is not responding to treatement.
- When regular blood sugar or other screening tests are not done.
- When the disease is present for a long period especially Type 1.

The complications which are commonly associated with diabetes are as follows:

Hypoglycemia or low blood sugar, ketoacidosis, heart disease, kidney disorders, eye complications, nerve complications, infections, gangrene of foot, and digestive system disorder.

Hypoglycemia or Low Blood Sugar

Hypoglycemia refers to the fall in blood sugar to the level of **50-60 mg/100ml or less**. It may be mild and self-limiting in patients of Type 2 Diabetes who are on oral medications. In contrast it can present as a serious emergency in Type 1 Diabetes patients who are on insulin injections.

The causes of low blood sugar in diabetic patients are summarized below:

- Due to a high dose of insulin injection or tablets.
- Due to error in calculating the dose.
- Starting with a higher dose in the early part of disease.

- Due to improvement in diabetes control.
- Due to reduced requirements after a stress is over or after an infection or delivery.
- When food is not taken immediately after injections or omitted completely.
- After severe exercise.
- In the presence of gastric, liver or kidney disease.
- If certain painkillers are taken along with oral medicines (tablets).
- In infants of diabetic mothers.

Features of Low-Blood Sugar

Features of low-blood sugar vary from patient to patient, with the adult experiencing symptoms earlier than children. The various features of the low-blood sugar are as follows:– increased appetite, vomiting sensation, sweating, feeling of weakness, tingling and numbness of lips and fingers, trembling, pounding heart, headache, blurring of vision or double vision, increased yawning, twitching of muscles, irritability or sadness or confusion or aggressive behaviour, and if not controlled or very severe, drowsiness, fits or loss of consciousness.

Diagnosis

- The diagnosis of this complication can be done by simple blood sugar estimation. It will reveal blood sugar level below 50mg/100ml. If some treatment is given before the blood sample is taken, the blood sugar level will be normal.
- The features of the disease and their disappearance immediately after treatment also clinch the diagnosis.
- Urine never contains sugar during this complication.

Treatment

Once hypoglycemia is suspected, the patient has to be given some carbohydrate containing food immediately and repeated once the blood sugar level report is available. Any of these substance may be given—a cube of sugar, 10-20 gm of glucose powder - Glucon-C, Glucon-D, Dextrose, Electral etc., fruit, bread, biscuit or Glucose in the liquid form may be given through the blood (by intravenous drip) depending on the seriousness of the situation.

- For complicated cases with fits, coma, abnormal behaviour, hospitalization is essential.

Prevention

- Patients and their relatives or guardians should learn to identify the warning symptoms of low blood sugar and act accordingly.
- They should report to their consulting doctors about these episodes and seek advice regarding change in dose or timing of medicines.

Patients should take their insulin injections or oral tablets just a few minutes before or during a meal.

If the meal is skipped or delayed for a long time low blood sugar will definitely occur.

- Oral medicines should never be taken along with alcoholic drink.
- If a strenuous exercise is done, it should be followed by some extra carbohydrate food item.
- All diabetic patients must carry an Identity card prepared by the Diabetes Association of India. It should contain name, address telephone number, doctor's name and address. The following appeal is normally written in the card:

"I am a diabetic patient.

If I am drowsy or behaving abnormally please give me sugar or sweet drink.

If I am unconscious please take me to a hospital or a doctor."

Along with this appeal the medicines and their doses are also given in the card.

The identity card saves the person's life in a case of emergency. Moreover many patients who develop low blood sugar and as a consequence exhibit abnormal behaviour, have been arrested on charges of being drunk and disorderly. Prolonged state of low blood sugar can permanently damage the brain.

Ketoacidosis

In uncontrolled diabetes due to deficiency of insulin, there is increased breakdown of fats leading to formation of ketone bodies in large quantities in blood and urine. Their elevated levels also lead to increased acidity of blood and tissues. Hence the term ketoacidosis.

Before the discovery of insulin, more than 50% of diabetic patients used to die due to ketoacidosis. Now less than 20% of diabetics in India die from Diabetic Ketoacidosis. The commonest cause of death is the ignorance on the part of patients and sometimes even the doctors to appreciate the danger signals of this complications arising out of uncontrolled disease.

Ketoacidosis is slightly more common in younger individuals especially of the fair sex and also those who are thin. It is also less common in India, Africa, Japan and West Indies probably due to low fat and high carbohydrate diets consumed in these countries.

The causes or provoking factors, which lead to this complication, are given below:

The patient omits or reduces the dose of insulin due to:

- Ignorance of its consequences.
- Non-availability of doctor for injecting the dose.
- Religious fasting or otherwise.
- Non-availability of food.
- Due to infections of the throat, lungs, skin, urinary system etc.
- Vomiting or diarrhoea due to dietary or other factors.
- Ineffective or inadequate dose of insulin injection.

- In newly diagnosed Type 1 diabetes patients as the first symptom.
- In stressful situations like pregnancy, injury, during an operation etc.

Features of the Disease

These are very few warning signals of this condition in the early phase of disease. Mostly the disease develops gradually except in the case of children. The common features of ketoacidosis are as follows: Intense thirst, passing increased volume of urine, vomiting, headache, loss of appetite, restlessness, weakness, pain in abdomen (cramps), constipation, drowsiness, and in late stage deep and rapid breathing, acidotic breath (odour of over ripe fruit), cool clammy skin, dry tongue, rapid and feeble pulse and ultimately coma.

Diagnosis

Besides the above features, a few laboratory test will confirm the diagnosis. The tests are as follows:

- Blood sugar levels are very high ranging upto 800mg/100ml or more.
- Urine contains sugar and ketone bodies.
- Blood is acidotic with low values of bicarbonate.

Treatment

The patient has to be urgently treated in the hospital. He may require the following:

- Insulin injections.
- Water and electrolytes replacement through venous blood (drip) to compensate water loss and acidity.
- Antibiotic injections to control infection.

Prevention

- Regular and timely intake of medicines and insulin.
- In case of stressful conditions and infections, dosage to be increased after consulting the doctor.

- If any unusual symptoms develop.
- Immediately inform the doctor.
- Take bed rest.
- Take plenty of fluids to prevent loss or deficiency of water and salts.
- If diagnosis is confirmed, patient has to be immediately rushed to hospital. If patient is already in coma, delay in treatment will make recovery very difficult.

Differences in coma due to low blood sugar and ketoacidosis is given in the table below:

Differences Between Coma due to Low Blood Sugar and Ketoacidosis

	Coma with low blood sugar	Coma with ketoacidosis
1.	Develops all of a sudden.	Develops after ill health for several days.
2.	Due to excessive dose of insulin injection.	Due to no insulin or less dose.
3.	Lack of food or missing meals.	Too much food intake.
4.	Increased appetite.	Decreased appetite.
5.	Abnormal behaviour.	Absent.
6.	Tingling and numbness of lips and fingers.	Absent.
7.	Heart beat normal.	Heart beat increased.
8.	Increased thirst and urination absent.	Present
9.	No acidotic or fruity odour of breath.	Present
10.	Breathing normal.	Increased breathing.
11.	Pulse is strong.	Pulse is weak.
12.	Abdominal pain and constipation absent.	Present.
13.	Urine does not contain glucose on ketone.	Urine contains glucose and ketone.
14.	Blood sugar levels low.	Blood sugar levels increased.
15.	Treatment by giving food	Treatment by insulin injections.

Diabetes and Heart Disease

Diabetic individuals are more prone to develop heart disease as compared to non-diabetic individuals.

The danger signals of heart disease in diabetics are easy fatigability (person gets tired easily), increased breathlessness on minimal exertion or even rest., chest pain in the centre or towards left side of chest, sudden uncontrolled blood sugar, and increase in the blood pressure.

Treatment of heart disease is always done in the hospital with regular monitoring of various body and laboratory parameters.

Prevention of Heart Disease in Diabetics

- Regular check-up of blood sugar and proper control with medicines.
- Monthly monitoring of blood pressure.
- Quarterly or half-yearly tests of heart function-ECG, blood tests.
- Prevent weight gain by promoting salt restricted, fat-free diet and regular exercise.
- A special test of fat content "Lipid Profile" if available may be done. It indicates the magnitude of risk of individual developing heart disease.
- Smoking and drinking of alcohol to be stopped.
- Oral pills in diabetic women to be used with caution.

Diabetes and Kidney Disorders

As in the case of heart, long-standing diabetes can also lead to complications in the kidneys. Patients with Type 1 Diabetes have 30-40% chance of developing kidney disorders after 20 years while it is 15-20% in Type 2, but since Diabetes Type 2 is more prevalent, kidney disease is more prevalent in Type 2 than Type 1.

In India 11% of deaths in diabetics are due to kidney disorders.

The mechanism of development of these disorders is same as that of the heart. There is deposition of fat on the walls of small and large blood vessels (arteries) of the kidney leading to narrowing of blood vessels and blood flow obstruction. Due to this defect, the blood pressure increases and waste products of the blood accumulate.

The danger signals of kidney disorders in diabetes are increased lassitude, breathlessness on exertion, increased urination at night, swelling of the ankle, unstable control of blood sugar (reduced insulin requirements), and increased blood pressure.

Diagnosis

- When kidneys are functionally normal, the urine contains no protein, while in diseased kidneys, urine contains protein which may rise upto 5gm in 24 hours or even more.
- When disease is advanced in stage, blood levels of urea and creatinine are very high.
- Due to diseased kidneys, urinary infection may develop as evidenced by pus cells and bacteria in urine.

Treatment

- Proper control of sugar by regular blood sugar monitoring and medicines.
- Treatment of high blood pressure if present.
- Treatment of urinary infection if present.
- In advanced disease of kidney, dialysis (removal of waste products from blood and re-circulation of purified blood) or kidney transplant may be required.

Prevention

Following measures in diabetics can prevent this disease:

- Regular monitoring of blood pressure and control whenever necessary.
- Regular monitoring of blood sugar and controlling it.
- Avoid medicines (e.g. painkillers, dyes for x-rays) which affect kidney function.

- Regular 24 hours urinary protein levels and blood tests for kidney function (blood urea and creatinine).

Complications of the Eye in Diabetes

When diabetes is present for a long time, the following complications of the eyes are likely to develop:
- Blindness due to damage to blood vessels of innermost part of eye-the retina.
- Cataract (Motia-Bind) or opacity of the lens of the eye.
- Myopia or short-sight where the person cannot see distant obejcts.
- Glaucoma (Kala-Motia) or increased pressure in the eye producing blurring of vision and sometimes blindness.

Blindness due to Retinal Damage

Diabetics have 25 times more risk of developing blindness than non-diabetics. After 10 years of diabetes 50% of patients develop blindness due to retinal damage which increases to 80% after 15 years.

About 10% of blind population in U.K. and U.S.A is diabetic.

Salient features of this disease are as follows: Patients with Type 1 and Type 2 diabetes are equally prone to develop this complication. The blindness is present in different age group and sexes. It may occur in one eye or both. Cause of blindness is reduced blood circulation in blood vessels of eyes due to increased fat deposition with resulting leakage of blood from friable (weak) vessels into the eye producing swelling and later blindness. In early part of the disease there is no symptom. In late disease patient complains of blurring of vision. The disease can only be diagnosed by examining the retina using an ophthalmoscope.

Treatment
- In early part of disease no treatment is required. By controlling blood sugar, blood pressure and reducing fat levels in blood, the disease can be totally controlled.
- In late part of disease treatment is by Laser Photocoagulation or by operation of the retina.

Prevention of Blindness in Diabetics

The blindness in diabetics can be prevented by the following measures:

- Eye examination every 6 months or 1 year after diabetes is diagnosed.
- Avoiding smoking or using tobacco in any form.
- Correction of high blood pressure by medicines and salt-restricted diet.
- Control of blood sugar by regular medicines and blood tests.
- Control of fat levels in blood by regular blood tests and fat-free diet.

Complications of the Nerves in Diabetes

Majority of patients with diabetes develop complications of the nerves. About 60% patients with about 25 years duration of diabetes are found to develop these complications though the number may increase upto 90% in many cases. These complications are detected in both Type 1 and Type 2 Diabetes and mainly in middle-aged or elderly individuals. Invariably they are seen in uncontrolled mild diabetes of long duration.

The nerves involved may be nerves of the hands and feet or those of the brain and spinal cord.

Causes of Damage to the Nerves

- Direct damage due to lack of carbohydrate metabolism.
- Due to reduced blood supply to the nerves.
- Due to deposition of fat in large and small arteries supplying the nerves of hands and feet or brain:

Symptoms of Nerve Damage in Diabetics

The spectrum of symptoms reported by patients with nerves complication are given below:

- Burning, cramp-like, piercing or dull aching pain in the feet and legs rarely in hand especially at night.

- Tingling, numbness or coolness in feet and legs followed by pain in muscles and insensitivity to hot, cold and pain sensations.
- Inability to maintain balance of body and strength and direction of movements of hands and feet.
- Deformities of toes and nails, thickened skin and ulcers on sole (due to insensitivity of feet to repeated injuries).
- Pain, weakness and thinning of muscles of thigh.
- Inability to control passing of urine.
- Repeated diarrhea or constipation.
- Abdominal cramps.
- Inability to sweat.
- Intolerance to extreme temperatures.
- Impotence.
- Fall in blood pressure on suddenly standing up from lying down position.
- Sudden attack of weakness or paralysis usually on one side of body (Stroke).
- Infections of the brain.

Diagnosis is made by nerves conduction studies (velocities) of affected nerves and Electromyography.

Treatment varies according to the presenting feature. Vitamins have no role in treatment.

Prevention

Proper evaluation of symptoms given above. Tests of nerve and muscles function as given above.

Infections

It is universally known that diabetes are very prone to develop infections of different types. About 8.5% of diabetic patients are known to die due to infections inspite of availability of various antibiotics.

The 3 major causes of infections are poor control of diabetes, reduced immunity or resistance to fight diseases, and defects in the blood vessels and nerves.

Types of Infections
- Urinary infections are commonest and increase during pregnancy.
- Chest infections like tuberculosis and pneumonia.
- Skin infection—Boils, carbuncles, fungal infections especially in the genital area in females.
- Rarely infections of bones and gall bladder.

Treatment involves control of blood sugar levels and proper antibiotics.

Gangrene of Foot

Gangrene refers to death or decay of a part of body.

Gangrene of the foot is very common in diabetes and has necessitated amputation (removal) of toes or even the whole foot in many cases.

Causes of gangrene destruction of nerves of the foot or lower limb are reduction in blood supply to the foot and skin infection of the foot or sole.

Symptoms of gangrene are initially pain in the foot affected, later loss of sensations in the foot, changes in the colour and texture, initially red then pale and finally black, coldness in the ankle and foot and skin infection of foot.

Treatment
- Controlling blood sugar is of utmost importance.
- Soft pad on the sole.
- Rest to the legs or complete bed rest.

- Treatment of infection with antibiotics.
- Treatment of pain with pain-killers.
- Amputation (removal) of affected toes or whole foot when disease is spreading or pain not controlled.

Prevention
- Regular monitoring of blood sugar.
- Examination of the feet yearly or twice a year.
- Washing feet daily and using lubricating creams, oils.
- Not to walk barefoot.
- Avoid extremes of temperature.
- Wear appropriately fitting shoes.
- Cut toe nails regularly.
- Never to cut corn or calluses.
- Treatment for skin diseases.

Digestive System Disorders

Some patients with diabetes may present with symptoms of digestive system due to nerve disturbances, which reduce movements of stomach and intestines or reduction in the blood supply or as a part of keto-acidosis.

Symptoms commonly reported are pain in the abdomen, vomiting, diarrhoea or constipation, loss of appetite, passage of smelling, fatty, sticky, stools and fullness of stomach after meals.

Treatment depends on the symptoms.

■ ■ ■

6. Diagnosis of Diabetes

he diagnosis of diabetes may appear to be simple and involve just demonstration of increased sugar levels in blood and sometimes in urine, but many facts and fallacies have to be understood.

Diabetes should be suspected in the following individuals:

Criteria for Suspicion of Diabetes

- In persons aged 40 years and above.
- With a history of diabetes in a blood relative.
- Excessively overweight.
- Persons with symptoms like increased thirst, appetite and loss of weight, inspite of good food intake, frequent infections, unexplained weakness.
- Persons with heart disease, high blood pressure or vague pains in the body.
- Women who have put on excessive weight during pregnancy.
- Women who have delivered a baby weighing more than 3.5kg.
- Multiple deaths of babies before or after birth.

The following tests are done to diagnose diabetes and to monitor progress of the disease with medicines.

Urine Examination

- Urine is examined for detection of glucose (sugar) and ketones.
- There are many tests, which are used for this purpose.

Benedicts' Test

This is the oldest test used to detect diabetes. It has of late become obsolete and is used only in remote primary health centres, where facilities for other tests are not available.

In a test-tube 8 drops of urine are mixed with 5ml (one teaspoonful) of Benedict's Qualitative Solution and boiled and colour noted. The results are interpreted as given below:

Results of Benedict's Test

Blue	Nil
Clear green	0.1%
Turbid green	0.3%
Green and yellow precipitate	0.5 to 1%
Yellow	1%
Orange	2%
Brick red	More than 2%

Fallacies of this Test

- It only gives a crude idea of diabetes, because it reveals presence of sugar only when blood sugar increases more than 180mg% i.e. in cases of severe diabetes.
- Even if other sugars i.e. fructose, galactose, maltose and lactose are found in urine, the test gives positive results.
- Certain medicines like aspirin, penicillin and other antibiotics and Vitamin C can also give positive results.
- In children collecting urine sample is difficult.

Dip-stick Methods

There are certain paper or plastic strips coated with chemicals that change colours according to sugar and ketone concentration. For example, one type of strip ranges from yellow through green to dark blue and another from blue through green to brown. The dip-stick is dipped in fresh urine or directly through the urine stream and within 30 seconds the reagent (chemical) side of paper is compared with corresponding colour chart given on the container. Various such dip-sticks are available in the market namely Diastix, Ketodiastix, Gluketur, Uristix etc.

Disadvantages

- It is costly, though cutting the strip longitudinally can reduce cost.
- Patients with colour blindness may misinterpret the results.
- Vitamin C and other medicines may interfere with the results.

The strips have a limited shelf life, especially after the container is opened.

Advantages

- It is a very simple procedure.
- Even the patient at home can do it.
- Result is instantaneous.
- It is useful for monitoring diabetes control at home. Patients with Type 1 Diabetes should check their urine samples 3 to 4 times a day and Type 2 once preferably 2 hours after a meal.

Tests for Ketones in Urine

Ketones in urine can be detected by following tests:

- Dip-stick Method—explained above
- Rothera's Test
- Gerhardt's Test

Blood Tests for Sugar (Glucose) Estimation

Diabetes can be accurately diagnosed by estimation of blood sugar.

The various tests, which are used, for estimating blood sugar are as follows:

Fasting Blood Sugar

After an overnight fasting of 10-14 hours, blood is taken from a vein or capillary (finger tip) and blood sugar is estimated using reagent kits by either.

- Enzyme-Linked-Immunosorbent Assay (ELISA) technique.
- Radio-Immunossay (RIA) technique.
- Dip-sticks similar to that used for urine examination.

Value of this Test

- This test alone cannot be used for diagnosing diabetes.
- In mild cases this test may be normal and diabetes may be missed.
- Reliability of this test is less because true fasting cannot be assured. People invariably make the mistake of having a cup of tea/coffee before the test.
- Normal fasting value of venous blood is 100mg% and a value more than 126mg% is mostly confirmatory of the disease.

Post-Prandial (P.P) Sugar

This test is based on the principle that after carbohydrate meal or glucose ingestion, blood sugar returns to fasting level within 2 to $2^1/_2$ hours.

The earliest evidence of carbohydrate tolerance to diabetes is a delay in the return of blood sugar values to fasting level.

This test is done 2 hours after a meal or after giving 75gm glucose powder in 300ml of water.

Value of this Test

- This is a better guide than fasting levels for diagnosing diabetes.
- Normal value is 200mg% and values above 200mg% indicates presence of diabetes.

- High values are seen in following conditions:

Prolonged inactivity, carbohydrate deprivation, excessive fat intake, liver disorder, menstrual period, advanced age and certain medicines like steroids, oral pills, sleeping pills.

- Low values are seen in following conditions:

    After exertion, vomiting, and aspirin.

    This test is also important for monitoring the control of diabetes.

If blood sample is taken 2 hours after a meal along with medicines for diabetes, the blood value gives an indication of control of the disease.

Random Blood Sugar

Random blood sugar estimation refers to the blood sample being taken at any particular time of the day especially when it does not correspond with a fasting or post-meal (prandial) state.

Value of this Test

This test only gives a very crude idea about the diabetes and has very little place in the diagnosis of diabetes.

It could be confirmatory only when values higher than 250mg% are found.

Glucose Tolerance Test (G.T.T)

Principle of this Test

This test is based on the principle that ingestion of glucose in a normal person leads to a rise in blood sugar level in $1/2$ to 1 hour and returns to fasting level within 2 to $2 1/2$ hours. In a diabetic the rise in blood sugar is greater, is sustained longer and there is a delay in returning to fasting levels.

Procedure

After an overnight fasting of 10-14 hours the person's blood is collected from a vein and repeated after 2 hours. In some cases the test may be prolonged to 3 to 4 hours. After taking the first sample in the fasting state, 75gm of glucose is dissolved in 300ml water and the test repeated every ½ hour for 2 hours.

This test should be done in a person on a normal diet and performing normal activities. During the test, the person must be at physical and mental rest and should not smoke. The values of this test in normal and diabetic individuals are given below.

G.T.T. Values for Normal and Diabetic Individuals

	Normal (mg%)	Borderline (mg%)	Diabetes (mg%)
Fasting	<110	110-125 (IFG)	> 126
After 2 hours	<140	140-199 (IGT)	≥ 200

NB: IFG – Impaired fasting glucose
IGT – Impaired glucose tolerance
These are intermediate stages of diabetes.

Value of this Test

- This test is a very useful one and gives almost fool proof diagnosis of diabetes.
- It is also useful in detecting borderline cases of diabetes that will eventually develop diabetes.
- It is not used these days because it is time-consuming and at times very ill, debilitated patients cannot undergo such a tedious test in a laboratory or hospital.
- Various factors affect the normal values of this test (Refer P.P. sugar).

Dextrometer/Glucometer

Certain portable devices are available which facilitate diagnosis and monitoring of diabetes in the doctor's clinic or even at home. Such devices are called as glucometer or dextrometer.

How to use Dextrometer/Glucometer

The person's blood is taken from the fingertip just one or two drops and applied to a tiny strip with a chemical coated pad at one end (Dextrostix, Hemoglukotest). This is then inserted into the dextrometer, which displays a digital reading of the blood sugar.

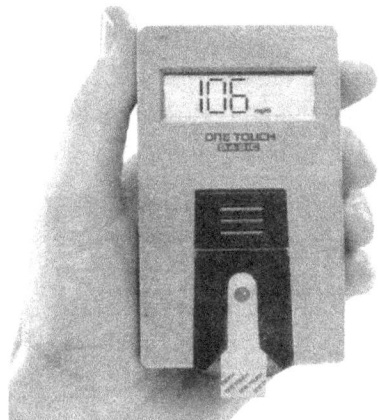

Fig. 6.1: Glucometer

Advantages and Disadvantages

This is a very reliable and a quick method of estimating blood sugar levels. This is especially useful for regular monitoring as in the case of newly diagnosed cases where dosage of medicines has to be adjusted initially. Patients with Type 1 and uncontrolled diabetes have to undergo blood tests 2-3 times a day and going to the laboratory several times a day may be difficult and time-consuming.

In cases of emergencies like low blood sugar and keto-acidosis especially and on holidays when the laboratory facilities are not available, this procedure becomes handy.

In elderly, bed-ridden patients and pregnant women who are not very mobile, the dextrometer is very useful.

Presently the dextrometer and the strips used are quite expensive, though cost may be reduced after import of various components is replaced by indigenous manufacture.

Glycosylated Haemoglobin

Haemoglobin is an iron containing substance found in our red blood cells and combines with oxygen and transports it to various body organs. Sometimes glucose gets attached to haemoglobin, the molecule being named glycosylated haemoglobin. The concentration of this glycosylated haemoglobin is a very good index of average glucose content in diabetics. It is higher in diabetic patients than normal individuals. Since each red blood cell has a life span of about 3 months, the value obtained gives an indication of blood glucose concentration of the past 3 months.

Value of this Test

- This is a very valuable test in diabetic pregnancy since it gives indication of metabolic control during pregnancy, which is important, since abnormal babies and death rate in foetuses can be minimized by proper sugar control.

- By knowing sugar control in last 3 months, modification in treatment can be done if necessary, thus long-term monitoring is possible.

- It is very useful for Insulin-dependent Diabetes where the fluctuation in blood-glucose is wide.

- Patient does not have to fast or go for test after a meal.

- It is not useful for diagnosing low-blood sugar or keto-acidosis.

- Day-to-day monitoring and treatment alteration is not possible.

- This can only by done in a good laboratory set-up.

- Unstable compound called pre-glycosylated haemoglobin can interfere with the results.

- In patients with anaemia, who have reduced haemoglobin and red blood cells, the value will be false.

- In patients with kidney com plications the values may be misleading.

Differences Between Urine and Blood Sugar Tests

Urine sugar tests	Blood sugar tests
1. Urine sugar is present only when blood sugar is more than 180 gm%.	Various values of blood sugar can be detected.
2. Useful only for diagnosing advanced diabetes.	Early and mild diabetes can even be diagnosed.
3. Other sugars (lactose, fructose etc.) may interfere and give positive sugar reactions.	Results not affected by other sugars.
4. Medicines like vitamin C, aspirin etc. may interfere with the results.	Do not interfere except when dipsticks are used.
5. In children collection of urine sample is difficult.	Collection of blood is painful but possible.
6. Emotional factors do not interfere during test.	May interfere during the test.
7. It is not an accurate method of monitoring.	It is an accurate method of monitoring diabetes control.

7. Treatment of Diabetes

Diabetes is a disease which is due to multiple contributory factors and it affects different systems of the body. Hence a multidisciplinary approach is required involving different modalities and systems of treatment for better and permanent results. This gives rise to better control of the disease, lesser complications and a prolonged life.

The Objectives of Treatment of Diabetes

- The patient should be relieved of almost all the symptoms.
- Attainment and maintenance of appropriate body weight to carry out daily routine.
- Glucose and fat levels in blood to be kept within normal limits.
- Various complications to be prevented or if present, to be treated with the best possible efforts.
- Regular check-up to know the efficacy of treatment.
- Side-effects of medicines be avoided or treated.
- Educate patients and relatives to undertake day to day management independently with the cooperation of the doctor.
- Patient should learn to live within the limits of the disease.
- Expert guidance required in special situations e.g. pregnancy, operations, accidents, sexual activity, travel etc.
- Patient should be able to lead a normal or near normal life in society.

Treatment Protocol

The approach to the treatment of Diabetes may be discussed under the following headings:

- Changes in the lifestyle
- Dietary management
- Role of physical exercise
- Role of Yoga
- Naturopathy
- Medical (Allopathic) treatment
- Ayurvedic remedies
- Magnetotherapy
- Acupressure
- Colour therapy
- Music therapy
- Feng Shui

Changes in the Lifestyle

The root cause of most cases of Diabetes is the erratic lifestyle of the affected individuals. The stress and tension of the modern life takes its toll on the health of individuals. Hectic office schedules, official deadlines and targets, family and social commitments affect the daily routine, dietary habits and sleeping patterns.

If the following changes are brought about in the lifestyle of individuals with Diabetes, they can bring about longlasting postive results:

- People with sedentary lifestyle can benefit remarkably by doing regular exercise and being active throughout the day.
- Stress can be overcome by practising yogasanas, pranayama, meditation and a postive attitude towards life.
- Smoking and consumption of tobacoo products like zarda, gutka, khaini should be given up completely.

- Excessive indulgence in tea, coffee, and alcohol should be given up completely or cut down drastically.
- As far as possible, all individuals should stick to a regular and disciplined daily routine with proper time to eat, sleep, work and attending to bowel habits.
- Those with obesity, sedentary lifestyle, stressful occupation or family history of diabetes should control their weight, diet, activity and attitude towards life.

Dietary Management

A well-planned and balanced diet is one of the major tools in the management of diabetes. The objectives of dietary treatment are given below:

- To maintain the blood sugar under sustained control.
- To lower the level of cholesterol and fat in the blood in obese individuals.
- To maintain an ideal weight.
- To balance the diet so that all nutrients are available at proper time.
- To enable the patient to live a normal span of life in health and comfort.
- To reduce medical treatment.
- To prevent long term complications e.g. heart attack, blindness, stroke etc.

Thus we can see that dietary treatment is not just meant for reducing the weight but there are many short and long-term objectives which play an important role in the managment of diabetes.

Diabetes is a chronic disease and so the diet, which is prescribed for the patients, should be of such a nature that it should suit the person in all aspects.

The Features of a Diabetic Diet

- It should be a mere modification of his usual diet.
- It should be very palatable.
- It should be a balanced diet.
- It should vary from day to day.
- It should be within the financial reach.
- It should be so spaced to avoid major fluctuations in blood sugar levels.
- The diet should not be different from that of other members of the family.
- It should be so simple that the patient and his spouse can understand it.

The important components of any diet are calories, carbohydrates, proteins, fats, vegetables and fruits and fibre.

Calories

Calories refer to the energy content of food. The requirements vary depending on the age, actual and expected body weight and nature of work. The table below shows calories requirement for different diabetics.

Calories Requirements for Different Diabetics

	Type of Diabetic	Kilocalories per day
1.	Labourer, Farmer	2600
2.	Young, hard working	2400
3.	Pregnant woman	2300
4.	Middle-aged, obese, sedentary	2000
5.	Middle-aged housewife	1700
6.	Elderly, sedentary person	1500
7.	Elderly obese person	1000-1200

Carbohydrates

Carbohydrates are mainly derived from cereals like rice or wheat, whichever is routinely used by the patient. Refined (simple) sugar e.g. sugar, honey, jams, cakes, pastries are totally prohibited because they produce sudden rise in blood sugar.

Requirements of carbohydrates in India is 150-300gm per day. Some nutritionists have advised the amount equal to $1/_{10}$ of total calories plus 30-50gm. The total carbohydrates required should be divided as 60% for the 3 major meals, 30% for 2-3 snacks and 10% for milk.

Proteins

The richest source of proteins is animal foods but actual intake of non-vegetarian food is restricted to once or twice a week in most Indian families due to the cost factor. Vegetable proteins in the form of pulses like bengal gram, green gram or black grams are more commonly consumed. Proteins of cereals and pulses have a supplementary effect and deficiency of one amino acid in one is made good by excess in other if taken together. Each meal should contain some amount of protein. Requirements for adults is 1 gm/kg/day and for children and pregnant and lactating women is 1.5-2 gm/kg/day.

Fats

Fat content of the diet is restricted to oils used in cooking, eggs and meat. At least 50% of fats should be in the form of polyunsaturated fattty acids (PUFA). Increased fat content leads to many complications like heart attack, stroke, blindness etc. Therefore blood levels of fats are to be checked regularly in diabetics and fat consumption in middle aged and elderly individuals are to be drastically reduced. Normal levels range from 180 to 250mg per 100ml of blood. Requirement of fats is usually 50-150 gm/day which is sufficient.

Vegetables and Fruits

Green leafy vegetables like spinach, cucumber, bitter gourd, cabbage, cauliflower, lady finger etc and fruits increase the bulk of the meals and satisfy patient's hunger without increasing the total calories. They also prevent constipation by increasing fibre content of diet.

Menu for Diabetics

The salient features of menu for diabetic patients are as follows:

- The menu should have breakfast, lunch, teatime snacks and dinner.
- For diabetics on long-acting Insulin there should be an evening snack at 5 p.m. and at bed time to prevent sudden fall of blood sugar.
- Diabetic children should have mid-morning snack.
- Meals should be reasonably uniform everyday.
- In patients receiving insulin injections, a delay or omission in meals is very dangerous.

Types of Diabetic Diet

The types of diabetic diet classified by nutritionists and dieticians are measured diabetic diet and unmeasured diabetic diet.

Measured Diabetic Diet

In this type of diet the exact quantities of foodstuffs to be taken are weighed. This is important for many middle-aged obese diabetics who have to lose weight in order to control the diabetes.

In such individuals high calorie foodstuffs e.g. rice, wheat flour, bread, pulses, oil, ghee, butter etc should be weighed. The size of utensils like katori (cup), spoon, plate and the size of chapati vary from one house to the other. Therefore, wheat flour, bread, rice etc should be weighed and rationed initially. Later the housewife can judge accurately even without weighing.

A sample of a measured diet of about 1500 Kilocalories is given below:

Bed Tea
1 cup tea or coffee (milk 30ml without sugar).

Breakfast
1 egg or paneer 30 gm.
1 slice bread or 2 chapattis (20 gm) or Idli.
1 cup milk (30ml without sugar).

Mid-morning Snacks
2 biscuits (sweet) or 4 salted biscuits or 1 fruit.
1 cup tea or coffee (30 ml milk without sugar).

Lunch
Dal (30gm) or paneer (35gm) or mutton (50gm) or chicken (70gm) or fish (100gm)
2 chapattis (20gm)
Mixed-vegetables (100 gm)
Curd (120 ml)
Salad (125 gm)

Tea
2 sweet biscuits or 4 salted biscuits or 1 fruit
1 cup tea or coffee (30 ml milk without sugar)

Dinner
Dal (30gm) or paneer (35gm) or mutton (50gm) or chicken (70gm) or fish (100gm)
2 chapattis (20 gm)
Mixed vegetables (100 gm)
Salad (125 gm)
Curd (120 gm)

Bed-time
200 ml milk

Other Important Points about Diabetic Diet:

- Special adjustments in diet are to be made in case of treatment with insulin injection, infections, diarrhoea, vomiting, social or religious gatherings, fasting etc.
- Patients with high blood pressure should also restrict their intake of salt.
- Eating while watching TV gives rise to increased calories intake.
- While going for shopping or on tour, special check has to be maintained on diet especially while eating outside.
- Eating when one is emotionally involved i.e. either happy, sad, angry or lonely can give rise to over or under-eating.

- People should not be carried away by food-fads and false beliefs of "hot foods", "cold foods" etc. When in doubt, consult a doctor or dietician.
- Sugar coated medicines, chewing gum, soft drinks, cough syrups, tonics etc. should be used with caution.

Follow the simplest rule in life: "WE EAT TO LIVE AND NOT LIVE TO EAT."

The diet can thus be adjusted depending on the calories intake requirements as follows:

- By increasing weight of wheat flour or bread slices.
- By increasing rationing of oil or ghee.
- By addition of butter.
- By changing skimmed milk to standard milk.
- By referring to the Calorie Reckoner of foodstuffs.

Calorie Reckoner of Foodstuffs
(Calories Relate to 100 gms, where Quantity not Specified)

Cereals and Cereal Products	Calories	Cereals and Cereal Products	Calories
Bajra	361	Dalia, Sweet	215
Cornflakes (25 gm)	95	Iddly 1 med.	100
Maize, flour	355	Macaroni (30 gm)	115
Maize, tender	125	Paratha, plain	275
Popcorn (50 gm)	170	Puri & potato	245
Ragi	328	Rawa appam	318
Rice, raw-milled	345	Rawa puttu	56
Rice, puffed	325	Uppma	230
Rice, cooked (60 gm)	70	*Pulses (Small)*	
Sago	351	Bengal-gram (roasted)	369
Suji	348	Green-gram, whole	334
Wheat flour (atta)	341	Lentil (masur)	343
Chapati (35 gm. atta)	119	Rajmah	346
Bread 1 slice	60	Soyabean	432
Bun	80	Bean sprouted	85
Oatmeal (27 gm)	110	Moong sprouted	60
Dosai, plain	130		

Cereals and Cereal Products	Calories	Cereals and Cereal Products	Calories
Chana Dhal	372	Egg 1 (40 gm)	65
Urad Dhal	347	Egg yolk 1	52
Dal (cooked) (92 gm)	92	Ham (cooked)	305
Rasam 1 cup	12	Lamb liver (raw)	136
Sambar 1/2 cup	105	Meat sausage	312
Sugars gur (15 gm)	57	Mutton (muscle)	194
Honey 1 teaspoonful	30	*Fishes*	
Jam (5 gm)	20	Anchovy (flesh)	165
Sugar 1 cube	12	Herring	106
Sugar (5 gm)	16	Hilsa	273
Fats and Oils		Katla	111
Butter (processed)	755	Lobster	90
Cream	213	Mrigal	98
Ghee (butter-fat)	900	Pomfret	87
Vegetables oil	900	Rahu	97
Margarine (sunbeam)	755	Sardines	80
Vanaspati (dalda)	900	Singhada	165
Milk and Milk Products		*Nuts*	
Milk, cow's 1 cup	100	Almonds (10 gm)	65
Milk, buffalo's 1 cup	115	Cashew-nuts (10 gm)	88
Milk, standardized 1 cup	137	Coconut (dry)	662
Milk, skimmed 1 cup	45	Coconut, tender	41
Milk, toned 1 cup	100	Ground-nuts	560
Milk, condensed 1 cup	320	Walnuts (15 gm)	102
Milk, powder	496	*Vegetables*	
Butter-milk, skimmed (1 glass)	25	Amaranth, chaulai	45
Chaina (cow's milk)	265	Channa-ka-sag	66
Cheese (amul)	348	Cabbage	45
Curds (cow's milk)	60	Arbi-ka-patta	56
Khoa (skim-buffalo's)	206	Fenugreek leaves (methi)	49
Custard (backed)	114	Mustard leaves (sarson)	34
Ice-cream	205	Radish leaves (mooli-ka-patta)	28
Kheer (Payasam)	178	Sarli Sag	86
Milk cake	331	Spinach (palak)	26
Cream	220	*Roots and Tubers*	
Paneer (100 gm)	100	Carrots (gajar)	48
Meat Products		Colocasia (arbi)	97
Bacon (raw)	405	Lotus root	53
Beef, muscle	114	Onion	50
Chicken (fryer)	109	Potato	97
Chicken (broiler)	151	Sweet potato	120

Cereals and Cereal Products	Calories
Tapioca	157
Turnip (shalgam)	29
Yam (zaminkand)	79
Other Vegetables	
Ash gourd (peta)	10
Bitter gourd (karela)	25
Bottle gourd (doodhi)	12
Brinjal	24
Broad beans	48
Cauliflower	30
Cardamom	229
Chillies, green	29
Chillies, dry	246
Cloves, dry	285
Coriander	288
French beans (phali)	26
Garlic, dry	145
Ginger, fresh	67
Jack fruit (kathal)	51
Ladyfingers (bhindi)	35
Mushrooms	42
Mogra	25
Amla	8
Papaya, green	27
Parmar (parmal)	20
Peas	93
Pepper, dry	304
Pepper, green	98
Plantain, green	64
Pumpkin (kaddu)	25
Tinda	21
Turmeric	349
Vegetable marrow-ghei	25
Water Chestnut (singhada)	115
Fresh Fruits	
Apple	56
Apricot	53
Banana	153
Rashbhari	53
Cherries	70
Dates	283

Cereals and Cereal Products	Calories
Figs	75
Guava	66
Grapes (blue)	45
Grape-fruit	32
Jamun	47
Lichis	61
Loquat	43
Malta	36
Mango	50-80
Melon-white	21
Water-melon	16
Mulberry	53
Orange	53
Papaya	32
Peaches	50
Pear	51
Pineapple	46
Plums	56
Pomegranate (red)	77
Sapota (cheeku)	94
Mausami	43
Dried Fruits	
Apricots	306
Dates, currants	317
Figs dried (20 gm)	55
Melon seeds	607
Raisins	315
Salads and Soups	
Beetroot	62
Cabbage	27
Carrots	48
Cucumber	13
Lettuce	21
Mint	48
Onion, (small)	59
Radish (white)	17
Radish (pink)	32
Tomato, (ripe)	21
Meat soup (150ml)	115
Chicken soup (150ml)	85
Vegetable soup (150ml)	12

Cereals and Cereal Products	Calories
Tomato cream soup (150ml)	85
Vegetable soup (1 cup)	65
Biscuits and Cakes	
Biscuit, salted 1	15
Biscuit, sweet 1	24
Arrowroot	20
Cheese-tid-bits (3.5 gm)	20
Coconut macaroon (13 gm)	80
Cake, chocolate, (45 gm)	165
Cake, fruit (30 gm)	117
Cake, plain (40 gm)	146
Snacks & Savouries	
Chakali (wheat flour)	550
Chat	474
Chewra (fried)	420
Dal Vadha 1 (30 gm)	200
Dhokla	122
Godam pongal	356
Mathi	420
Meat puff (50 gm)	200
Muruku	521
Namakpara	583
Pakora	200
Potato chips (20 gm)	110
Potato kachori	166
Rawa adai	326
Samosa	256
Tapioca chips	570
Aloo vada	118
Cutlet	125
Tomatos sandwich	180
Papad (fried)	43
Padad (grilled)	25
Sweets	
Badam halwa	570
Balushahi	469
Burfi (25 gm)	100
Fruit jelly	75
Gujia	500
Gulab jamun (25 gm)	100

Cereals and Cereal Products	Calories
Imarti (40 gm)	200
Jalebi	412
Kalkai	350
Mysore pak	357
Nankhatai	584
Petha (50 gm)	83
Pinni	490
Rasgula (30 gm)	100
Shakarpara	570
Sohan Halwa	400
Suji Halwa	136
Sweet appam	250
Sweet Kolkattai	194
Yela Adai	232
Sandesh	57
Beverages: Soft & Alcoholic	
Apple juice (200 ml)	95
Coconut water, (200 ml)	50
Orange juice (200 ml)	95
Tea (with 1 oz milk, no sugar)	22
Coffee (with 1 oz milk, no sugar)	25
Gingeraly 1 bottle	60
Coke 1 bottle	80
Limca 1 bottle	50
Grape fruit juice (200 ml)	65
Tomato Juice (200 ml)	45
Beer (240 ml)	112
Brandy (30 ml)	73
Gin (dry) (43 ml)	105
Rum, whisky (43 ml)	105
Sherry (60 ml)	84
Wines (port) (100 ml)	160
Miscellaneous	
Horlicks (10 gm)	41
Ovaltine/Bournvita (10 gm)	38
Pickles (20 gm)	
(a) Mango sour	65
(b) Vegetable sweet	40
Tamarind pulp	283

Unmeasured Diabetic Diet

Patients who are mildly obese or of normal weight or those who are unable to measure their diet, the unmeasured diet is used. It mainly refers to list of food-items, which are categorized into 3 groups.

- Food items to be avoided altogether, mainly simple sugars and fatty foodstuffs.
- Food items to be eaten in moderate amounts.
- Food items to be eaten as desired.

Food Items to be Avoided Altogether

- Sugar/glucose, jaggery.
- Jam, jelly.
- Marmalade.
- Honey.
- Tinned fruits and fruit juices.
- Sweets, chocolates.
- Lemonade and other sweetened soft drinks like Campa-Cola, Limca etc.
- Cakes and pastries.
- Sweet biscuits.
- Pies, puddings.
- Sauces.
- Cream and cream cheese.
- Condensed milk.
- Sweetened desserts.
- Fried food like paranthas, samosas.
- Ice cream, kulfi and candy.
- Wines and beer.
- Butter, ghee.

Food Items to be Eaten in Moderate Amounts

- All types of bread.
- Rolls, scones, crisp breads.

- Potatoes, sweet potatoes, colocasia (arbi), yam.
- Peas and baked beans.
- Breakfast cereals.
- Fresh or dried fruits*, nuts.
- Macaroni, custard and foods with much flour.
- Diabetic foods.
- Milk (full cream).
- Polished white rice.
- Wheat or bajra preparations, suji, maida, sago, arrowroot.

Food Items to be Eaten as Desired

- Meat, fish, eggs (non-fried).
- Cheese.
- Tomato or lemon juice.
- Tea or coffee (without sugar).
- All vegetables especially green leafy ones (Bittergourd, frenchbeans, brinjals, ladyfinger, cabbage, kakri, soyabeans, drumsticks).
- Spices, salt, pepper and mustard.
- Saccharine preparations.
- Wheat flour with bran, brown rice or rice without starch water.
- Skimmed milk.
- Less sweet fruits like guava, papaya, jamun, phalsa, aroo, apple, orange.

Role of Physical Exercise

In addition to dietary treatment physical exercise plays an important role in the management of diabetes. Exercise is an important part of the treatment programme both for Type 1 Diabetes (who are underweight) and Type 2 Diabetes (who are overweight) patients. A

---

* Fruits with high sugar content like banana, chiku, grapes, lichees, mango, anaar and mausambi.

person is considered to be overweight or obese based on his Body Mass Index which is calculated as follows:

Body Mass Index (BMI) = Weight (kg) / Height (Meter)^2

Men are considered to be obese or overweight if their BMI is more than 30 and women if their BMI is more than 28.6.

The BMI of an individual can be calculated from his height and weight. The desirable weight ranges and the weight, which consider an individual obese are given in the table below:

For example if a man whose height is 1.60 mt (5'4") and weight is 78kg his BMI=78/(1.6x 1.6) = 30.5 which means that he is obese.

If his weight were to be 65 kg, his BMI = 65 / (1.6 x 1.6) = 25.4 which is normal for his height.

Weights of Normal and Obese Indian Men and Women

Height (without Shoes) (Metre/Feet)	Men Desirable Weight Range (kilograms)	Obese (kg)	Women Desirables Weight Range	Obese (kg)
1.45 (4ft 10")			42-53	64
1.48 (4ft 11")			42-54	65
1.50 (5ft)			43-55	66
1.52 (5ft 1/2")			44-57	68
1.54 (5ft 1")			44-58	70
1.56 (5ft 2")			45-58	70
1.58 (5ft 3")	51-64	77	46-59	71
1.60 (5ft 4")	52-65	78	48-61	73
1.62 (5ft 5")	53-66	79	49-62	74
1.64 (5ft 5 1/2")	54-67	80	50-64	77
1.66 (5ft 6")	55-69	83	51-65	78
1.68 (5ft 7")	56-71	85	52-66	79
1.70 (5ft 8")	58-73	88	53-67	80
1.72 (5ft 9")	59-74	89	55-69	83
1.74 (5ft 10")	60-75	90	56-70	84
1.76 (5ft 10 1/2")	62-77	92	58-72	86
1.78 (5ft 11")	64-79	95	59-74	89
1.80 (6ft)	65-80	96		
1.82 (6ft 1")	66-82	98		
1.84 (6ft 2")	67-84	101		
1.86 (6ft 2 1/2")	69-86	103		
1.88 (6ft 3")	71-88	106		
1.90 (6ft 4")	73-90	108		
1.92 (6ft 5")	75-93	112		

Benefits of Exercise

Weight Reduction

The most important benefit derived from exercise is the reduction in weight of the body. This is especially important for patients with Type 2 Diabetes who are obese. It has been observed that many of such patients revert to normalcy i.e. diabetes is cured after they have lost sufficient weight to attain the desirable weight. The mechanism of this change is the increase in the number of insulin receptors on losing weight. This increase is very effective in controlling diabetes.

Increased Efficacy of Insulin

Besides the control in weight, regular physical exercise can increase the efficacy of insulin in lowering blood sugar and supplying glucose to the body. In patients with Type 1 Diabetes where there is complete deficiency of insulin, exercise reduces the requirement of insulin by increasing the sensitivity of body to insulin. In Type 2 Diabetes where very little insulin is available in the pancreas exercise can increase the effectiveness of whatever insulin is available in the body. It has been observed that obese individuals have very few receptors attached to their cells as compared to those with normal weight. Due to the reduction in the number of receptors the cells which require regular supply of glucose for their normal activities are not able to respond to the available insulin in the body. This gives rise to surplus (excess) sugar (glucose) content in the blood i.e. diabetes. When the obese individuals lose weight, the number of such insulin receptors increase and hence each and every cell gets its regular quota of glucose and also the blood level of glucose normalizes. Thus losing weight means to control or even cure diabetes.

Reduced Risk for Heart Disease

Diabetes is associated with the long-term complication of heart disease due to deposition of fat in the blood vessels that decrease the blood circulation and gives rise to heart attacks. Exercise protects the heart by improving the efficiency of heart to pump blood as well as by increasing levels of certain protective elements known as High-Density Lipoproteins (HDL's) in the blood. These HDLs are known two indirectly decrease the fat (cholesterol) content in blood and improve the blood circulation

Normalization of Blood Pressure

It is well known that high blood pressure is associated with diabetes. Exercise normalizes the blood pressure by improving the circulation of blood in the heart and kidneys by preventing deposition of fat in the blood vessels.

Improvement in the Sense of Well-being

By reducing physical and mental tensions and strains, exercise improves the patient's sense of well being. Patient feels active, comfortable and cheerful after regular exercise.

Reduced Consumption of Medicines and their Costs

Exercise indirectly reduces the requirements of medicines, both tablets and injections due to improvement in diabetes control. This also reduces the exorbitant expenses incurred on medicines.

Types of Exercises

Every diabetic has to be evaluated in terms of the type of exercise he has to undertake by the treating physician. An Electrocardiogram (ECG) is done while putting in the person to exercise stress and his heart rate is evaluated. This heart rate should not exceed 70% of target rate (220 beats per minute minus age). For example a 50-year-old diabetic should not develop a heart rate of more than 119 beats/minute while doing exercise. Thus it can be decided as to what type of exercise the person should undertake. Generally exercises may be graded as mild, moderate or severe as follows:

Mild—Walking, household chores, cycling, gardening, boating, jogging, golf.

Moderate—Swimming, cricket (bowling), badminton, volleyball, table tennis, roller-skating, horse-riding.

Severe—Tennis, squash, running (16 mph), ice-skating, sking, and mountan climbing.

Frequency and Timing of Exercise

Exercise if done regularly can bring about conditioning of the heart i.e. the heart works less hard to do a job than before. This prevents heart attacks and keeps the person fit and fresh throughout the day. If regular exercise is not done, the benefit derived earlier is lost. Thus exercise should be done at least thrice a week i.e. every alternate day. The intensity of exercise should be such that the heart rate never exceeds the target rate. Exercise should be done for at least 30 minutes in each session. Warming-up and cooling down before and after exercise is also important. Brisk-walking and jogging is claimed to be the best and safest form of exercise. The best time to do exercise has been claimed to be 15-30 minutes after a meal. This is believed to be an ideal time because the blood sugar levels are at the peak during this time and chances of developing low blood sugar levels are remote provided the exercise is not done for more than two hours. This is especially important for patients on insulin injections are prone to develop low blood sugar levels. Such individuals should never undertake dangerous sports like scuba diving, parachuting, ice skating etc. Exercise during illness, extreme weather conditions is not advisable and if essential, a family member should accompany them to prevent low blood sugar levels.

Role of Yoga

Yoga is an ancient Indian technique of intergrating human personality at the physical, mental, moral and spiritual levels.

Maharishi Patanjali defined Yoga as "Chitta Vritti Nirodha" or control of mind and its fluctuations. He described eight aspects of Yoga which may be used to attain a healthy, happy and spiritual life. These are as follows:

- "Yama" or moral principles like non-violence, truth fulness, honesty, celibacy and covetousness.
- "Niyama" or rules of discipline like purity, contentment, austerity, introspection and dedication to God.
- "Asanas" or Yogic postures.
- "Pranayama" or control of breathing.
- "Pratyhara" or control of mind and sense organs.
- "Dharana" or concentration.
- "Dhyana" or meditation.
- "Samadhi" or a state of transcendental consciousness when the individual merges with the universal spirit.

From the treatment point of view Yoga can be divided as follows:

- Yogasanas
- Yogic Kriyas
- Pranayama
- Meditation

Yogasanas

Yogasanas refer to the yogic postures of the body which help in the physical, mental and spiritual development of the individual.

There are many differences between physical exercise and Yogasanas. These are highlighted in the table below:

Differences Between Physical Exercise & Yogasanas

		Physical Exercise	Yogasanas
1.	Movement of body	Moves rapidly.	Moves slowly and uniformly.
2.	Age groups	Restrictions are present in different age groups especially older people.	Can be practised by male, female and aged persons.
3.	Good effect on body	Strengthens the muscles.	Strengthens the mind and also the muscles.
4.	Outcome	Causes anxiety, exhaustion & weariness.	Tone up the nerves and internal organs of body. Exhaustion & weariness not felt.
5.	Development of body & mind	Mainly assists in development of body.	Develop, body, mind & prana.
6.	Flexibility of body	Lesser	More
7.	Discontinuation	Cannot be given up suddenly.	Can be discontinued at any time.
8.	Diet	Very rich food is required.	Simple and pure food.
9.	Prevention & cure of diseases	Prevention possible. Cure not available.	Have such powers.

How do Yogasanas Help in the Treatment of Diabetes

- All abdominal organs including the pancreas are toned up and the digestion and metabolism of food substances are enhanced.
- By improving the metabolism, blood levels of fat and sugar are reduced.
- There is a proper conditioning and rejuvenation of the neuro-endocrine (hormonal) system enhancing the effect of insulin and other hormones.
- The immune system is activated enabling the body to withstand greater stress, strain including that due to diseases.
- Accumulated toxic substances and excretory products are easily eliminated keeping the body fit, strong and rejuvenated.
- Regular practice of Yogasanas help to voluntarily control the heart rate, respiration, excretion, body temperature, requirement of food, sleep etc. bringing about a state of economical self-preservation and conservation of energy.

Yogasanas Useful for Treatment of Diabetes

Certain asanas are very useful in the treatment of Diabetes. These are Dhanurasana, Paschimottanasana, Sarvangasana, Halasana, Bhujangasana, Ardhamatsyendrasana, Matsyasana, Shashankasana, Pawan Muktasana, Chakrasana, Salavasana, and Mayurasana.

Detailed description of certain important asanas are given below:

Dhanurasana or Bow Pose

Techniques

- Lie down in the prone position (on the stomach) with the face and forehead touching the ground with the legs straight and the arms by the side.
- Exhale and bend the legs at the knee and hold them firmly by the hands at the ankles on the same side.
- Inhale, raise the thighs, chest and head simultaneously.

- The weight of the body should be on the navel and the head should be raised as high as possible with eyes looking upwards.

- This posture should be held as long as it is felt comfortable.

- Some authors recommend mild rocking movement on the abdomen, which bears the weight.

- Repeat this three to five times.

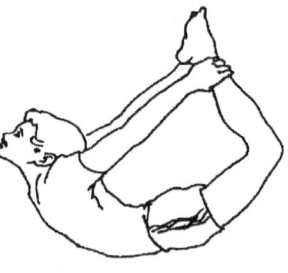

Fig. 7.1: Dhanurasana

Precautions

- This asana should not be done by those suffering from high blood pressure, slipped disc, hernia, colitis, duodenal ulcer and heart diseases.

Paschimottanasana (Back Stretching Pose)
Techniques

- Sit on the floor with the legs outstretched, feet together and hands on the knees.

- Relaxing the whole body slowly bend forward from the hips, sliding the hands down the legs. Try to grasp the big toes with the fingers and thumbs. If not possible hold the heels, ankles or any part of the legs that can be reached comfortably.

- Hold this position for a few seconds.

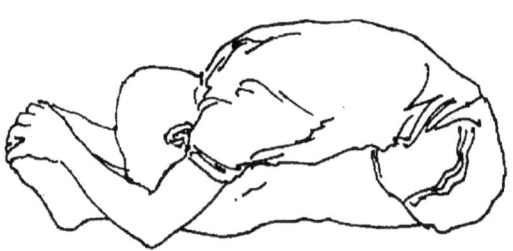

Fig. 7.2: Paschimottanasana

- Keep the legs straight, bend the elbows and gently bring the trunk down towards the legs keeping a firm grip on the toes, feet or legs. Touch the knees with the forehead and hold in this position as long as it is comfortable.
- Slowly return to the original position.
- Relax and repeat the exercise 2 to 3 times.

Precautions
- People who suffer from slipped disc lumbar spondylitis or sciatica should not perform this asana.
- Similarly those with cardiac problems, hernia and those who have undergone abdominal surgery should avoid this asana.

Sarvangasana or Shoulder Stand
It is a core exercise for all practitioners of Yoga and sometimes called as "the mother of all asanas".

Techniques
- Lie down in a supine position with legs and arms straight, feet together and palms facing downward.
- Take a deep breath and lift both the legs slowly upwards till they are at right angle to the body.
- After exhaling pause for a few seconds.
- Inhale and lift legs, buttocks and lower back with the forearms so that the chin presses into the sternum. Thus the entire weight of the body rests on the head , neck and shoulders and the arms are used for balancing.
- Focus the eyes on the big toes with the chin pressed against the chest and breathe slowly.
- Maintain this posture for 2-3 minutes.

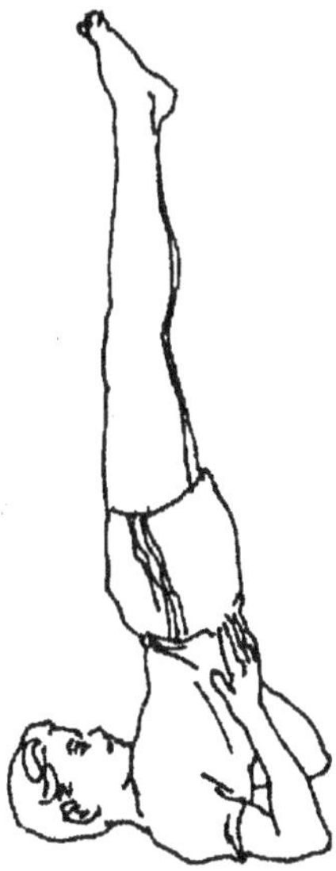

Fig. 7.3: Sarvangasana

- Exhale and bring down the legs after releasing the hands and the palms.

Precautions

- This asana should not be practised by individuals with high blood pressure, heart disease, cervical spondylitis and slipped disc.
- Obese individuals, people with a weak backbone or abdominal muscles and beginners are advised to support their legs against a wall initially.
- It should be avoided during menstruation and advance pregnancy.

Bhujangasana (Serpent Pose)

Techniques

- Lie flat on the ground in the prone position with legs straight and feet extended, touching each other and forehead pressed to the ground.
- Breathe in, press the head back and slowly raise the head and shoulders off the ground by bending the neck and back muscles.
- Keeping the arms straight, lift the abdomen above the navel from the ground with the head looking upwards into the sky.
- Hold your breath and remain in the posture for a few seconds with the weight of body balanced by the arms.
- Slowly exhale and come back to original position. Repeat the process 2-3 times.

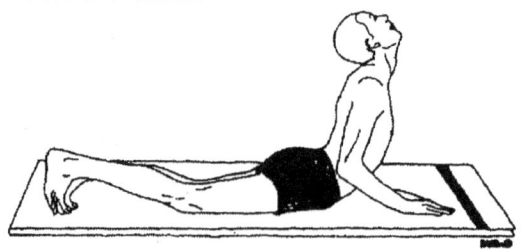

Fig. 7.4: Bhujangasana

Precautions
- Individuals who suffer from hypertension, Peptic ulcer, hernia, intestinal TB, and hyperthyroidism should not practise this asana.

Ardhamatsyendrasana (The Spinal Twist Pose)
This asana is a very important one since it strengthens the flexibility of spine laterally (sideways) which no other asana can accomplish. It is a very useful asana for diabetes patients.

Techniques
- Sit on the floor with the legs extended in front and feet together.
- Bend the right knee and bring the heel of the right foot close to the left buttock.
- Now bend the left knee and place the foot on the outer surface of the right knee.
- Turn the trunk and face towards the left shoulder placing the left arm behind the back.
- Hold the left ankle with the right hand.
- Try to hold the left leg with the left hand.
- Some authors advise bringing the right hand under the left knee and joining the palm of the left hand.
- Remain in the final pose for a few seconds and then return to the original position.
- Repeat the same with the other side.

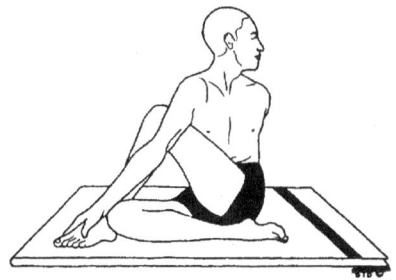

Fig 7.5 : Ardhamatsyendrasana

Precautions
- This asana should be done slowly and steadily without exerting undue pressure on the spine.
- People with peptic ulcer, hernia, hyperthyroidism, sciatica, and pregnant women, should practise this asana only under expert guidance.

Yogic Kriyas

Yogic Kriyas are a very important part of Hatha Yoga as they help to eliminate the accumulated toxins from the body. The body is like a machine which has to be continuously cleaned and maintained in a perfect condition. The Yogic Kriyas are six in number and often referred to as Shat Kriyas. They are as follows:

- Neti
- Kapalbhati
- Dhauti
- Nauli
- Basti
- Trataka

Kriyas useful for treatment of diabetes are Kapalbhati, Vaman Dhauti or Kunjal Kriya, and Nauli.

Kapalbhati (Frontal Brain Cleansing)

Kapalbhati is basically a technique of pranayama though older yogic texts have classified it as a part of Shatkarmas. It is of three types: Vatkrama Kapalbhati, Vyutkrama Kapalbhati and Sheetkrama Kapalbhati.

Vatkrama Kapalbhati

This is the most useful technique for treatment of diabetes.

Techniques
- Sit in any comfortable asana with the head and spine straight and the hands resting on the knees.

- Close the eyes and relax the whole body.
- Inhale deeply through both nostrils expanding the abdomen and exhale with a forceful contraction of the abdominal muscles, making a hissing noise.
- The next inhalation takes place by passively allowing the abdominal muscles to expand spontaneously without any effort.
- After completing 10 rapid breaths in succession, inhale and exhale deeply completing one round.
- Complete 3 to 5 such rounds.

Precautions
- The rapid breathing in this technique should be from the abdomen and not from the chest.
- It should be practised after asanas or Neti and preferably on an empty stomach or 3 to 4 hours after meals.
- If pain or giddiness is experienced, it should be stopped for a while and continued.
- Kapalbhati should not be practised by those suffering from heart disease, high blood pressure, vertigo, epilepsy, stroke, hernia or peptic ulcer.

Vaman Dhauti or Kunjal Kriya
Techniques
- Take about 1 litre of lukewarm water flavoured with aniseed and cardamom, to which some salt is added.
- Drink this water as quickly as possible till a vomiting sensation is felt.
- Stand up immediately, bend forward and insert first 3 fingers of the right hand into the mouth and tickle the uvula till vomiting is induced.

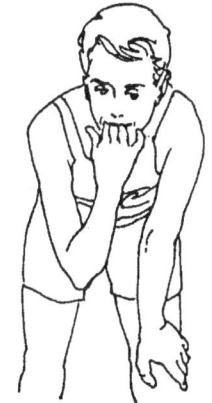

Fig. 7.6: Kunjal Kriya or Vaman Dhauti

- Continue this process till all the water comes out.
- This can be repeated once a week.

Precautions
- This procedure should be done in the early morning on an empty stomach.
- Food should not be taken for at least half an hour after practice.
- Finger nails should be trimmed well and hands washed with soap and water before performing the procedure.
- Persons suffering from stomach ulcers, eye diseases, heart problems, stroke, hernia should avoid this kriya.

Nauli
It is a Yogic kriya of massaging the whole abdomen and stomach by contracting and rolling the abdominal muscles, especially the rectus abdominis muscle.

Techniques
- Stand erect with feet about half a metre apart.
- Lean forward and place the hand on both thighs just above the knees.
- Inhale deeply holding the breath inside and bend the head forward and downward. Press the chin tightly into the sternum and pull the shoulders up and forward (Jalandhar Bandh).
- Exhale deeply, raise the diaphragm and chest, flattening the abdominal wall against the spine forming a hollow cavity (Uddiyana Bandh).
- Press the thighs with both hands until the rectus abdominis muscle is thrust out prominently in the centre of hollow abdomen. This is Stage I or Madhyamna Nauli.
- Now bring the rectus abdominis muscles at the left side of the abdomen by pressing hard the left thigh with the left hand. This is Stage II or Vama Nauli.

- Similarly bring the rectus abdominis muscle at the right side of the abdomen. This is Stage III or Dakshina Nauli.
- Now try to roll the rectus abdominis muscles so that they move from left to right with the breath held still.
- Then inhale, relax, and after normal respiration repeat the process of rolling the muscle from right to left.

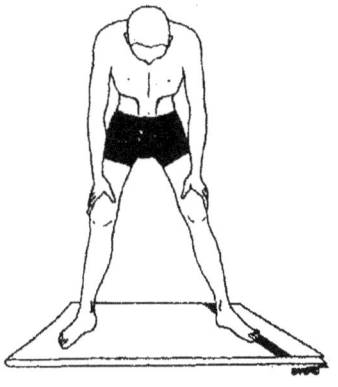

Fig. 7.7: Nauli

Precautions
Nauli should not be attempted by people suffering from heart disease, hypertension, hernia, gallstones, peptic ulcer, after abdominal surgery and during pregnancy.

Pranayama

Definition
Pranayama is derived from two sanskrit words – "Prana" and "Ayama". "Prana" means breath, life, vitality, air, power or energy. "Ayama" denotes extension, abstinence, regulation, control or restraint. Thus Pranayama is the act of control of respiration and an attempt to control the flow of "Prana" or vital force in the human body.

Stages of Pranayama
Pranayama consists of four stages:

- The "Puraka" or Inhalation Phase: Long, slowly controlled and sustained flow of inhalation.
- The "Kumbhaka" or Breath-holding phase: Controlled suspension and retention of breath after inhalation.
- The "Rechaka" or Exhalation Phase: Long, slow and controlled exhalation.

- "Shunyaka" or End of Breathing: Breath holding after exhalation.

Rules for Pranayama

- Pranayama is to be preferably practised in the open air or in a quiet, clean, well-ventilated room.
- The best & most comfortable posture for pranayama is padmasana.
- The place for such a practice is to be neat & clean and without any distractions.
- Pranayama should not be practised at a crowded place where pure air is not available. It may be done on a river bank.
- The best time for Pranayama is early morning when the air is pure and oxygen is available. If not possible it may be done in the evening after sunset.
- Tight dress should not be used, but loose comfortable clothes.
- One should not smoke at least 1 hr. before or after practice.
- Pranayama should be done under the guidance of an expert.
- After a night's good rest, it should be done.
- Breathing should be done through the nostrils only.
- The breath-holding practice should not be done by heavy weight lifters.
- Pranayama should not be practised while walking or lying.
- There should be a gap of at least 3 hrs. between taking of medicine & beginning of pranayama.
- If one feels dizzy while practising pranayama it may be due to excess practice or wrong practice.
- Pranayama should be practised after asanas and before meditation.
- A bath may be taken before commencing the practice or at least the hands, face and feet may be washed. After pranayama, the bath should not be taken for at least half an hour to allow the body temperature to normalize.

- Pranayama should be done on a empty stomach or three to four hours after a meal.
- No undue strain should be applied as lungs are very delicate organs and can be easily injured.
- Some individuals may exhibit certain symptoms while practising pranayama i.e. itching, tingling, heat or cold, feeling of heaviness, constipation or reduced urination. These symptoms usually disappear with regular practice. If persistent, a yoga expert may be consulted.

Benefits of Pranayama
- Pranayama improves the function of the lungs by increased oxygenation of blood vessels of the lungs as well as all parts of the lungs.
- Is increases the capacity of the lungs to inhale and exhale air.
- Breath-holding can train the body to tolerate low oxygen levels as seen while climbing the mountains.
- The blood supply to the heart and brain is improved by Pranayama.
- It enhances the concentration of mind and improves the relaxation of the body.
- Pranayama cleans up and purifies the nose, nasal sinuses and respiratory passages.
- The digestion is improved due to improved blood supply and pressure of the diaphragm on the abdominal organs. In Diabetes the pancreatic function is rejuvenated and toxic substances removed from digestive tract.
- Plavini Pranayama is believed to exert control over hunger and thirst in the individual who practises it.

Pranayama Useful for Treatment of Diabetes
Nadi Shodhana Pranayama, Bhastrika, Sheetali, and Sheetakari.

Nadi Shodhana Pranayama or Anuloma-Viloma
Techniques

- Sit in any comfortable meditative posture preferably padmasana keeping the head and spine upright.
- Close the eyes, relax the body and breathe freely for some time.
- Rest the index and middle fingers gently in the centre of eyebrows and the thumb and ring finger above the right and left nostrils respectively. These two fingers control the flow of breath in the nostrils by alternately pressing on one nostril and blocking the flow of breath and then the other. This is the Nasikagra Mudra.

Step – I

- Close the right nostril with the thumb and breathe in through the left nostril, mentally counting 1,2,3. Similarly close the left nostril with the ring finger, releasing pressure of thumb on the right nostril and breathe out, mentally counting 1,2,3. The time for inhalation and exhalation should be equal.
- Repeat the procedure by inhaling through the right nostril and exhaling though the left one. This makes up one round. Ten rounds are to be practised.
- Slowly increase the counting up 12:12 for inhalation/exhalation. This is followed by changing the ratio to 1:2 i.e. breathe in for count 5 and breathe out for count 10 adding upto ratio 12:24.

Step – II

After mastering step I , this step should be practised.

- Close the right nostril and inhale through the left nostril for a count of 5. After this close both nostrils and retain air in the lungs for a count of 5. Then, open the right nostril, breathe in slightly and slowly breathe out for a count of 5.
- This is repeated by inhaling from the right nostril, retaining and breathing out from the left side. Repeat 10 rounds.

- Increase the ratio from 1 : 1: 1 for inhalation, retention and exhalation to 1 :1:2, then 1:2:2, 1:3:2 and 1:4:2.

Step –III

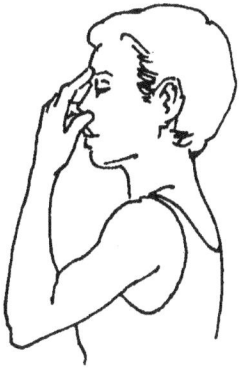

- In this step, inhalation is started from the left nostril as above, followed by retention (breath-holding) and exhalation from right nostril which is also followed by breath-holding.

- The procedure is also repeated as above by inhalation from the right nostril and 10 rounds are completed.

- The ratio is started as above 1:1:1:1 and increased to 1:4:2:2 and duration is also increased from a count of 5 to the maximum limit where comfortable..

Fig. 7.8: Nadi Shodhana Pranayama

Precautions

- Breathing should be free flowing and never forced.
- Breathing should never be done through the mouth.
- This technique of Pranayama is best done under the guidance of an expert.
- If there is any sign of discomfort, the procedure should be discontinued.
- The best time to practise is early in the morning after the asanas.
- The duration of this pranayama should be about 10 to 15 minutes daily comprising 5 to 10 rounds.
- Patients suffering from hypertension and heart disease must avoid breath-holding in this pranayama.

Bhastrika Pranayama

Techniques

- Sit in any comfortable meditative posture with hands resting on the knees in Gyana Mudra.
- Keep the head and spine straight, close the eyes and relax the whole body.
- Using Nasikagra Mudra close the right nostril with the thumb.
- Breathe in and out forcefully, without straining through the left nostril about 10 times. The abdomen should expand and contract rhythmically with the breath.
- Now close the left nostril and breathe rapidly and forcefully through the right nostril.
- Similarly breathing can be done through both the nostrils simultaneously.
- At the end of each procedure, breath-holding may be done for upto 30 seconds.

Precautions

- During Bhastrika only the abdomen should move and not the chest or shoulders.
- The breathing sound should only appear from the abdomen and not the throat or chest.
- If there is a feeling of giddiness, vomiting or excessive perspiration, the pranayama should be stopped.
- Violent respiration, facial contortions and excessive shaking of the body should be avoided.
- Bhastrika should not be practised by people suffering from hypertension, heart disease, duodenal ulcer, hernia, stroke, epilepsy or vertigo.
- Neti may be practised if there is blockage of nostrils with mucus.

Sheetali Pranayama
Techniques
- Sit in any comfortable meditation posture with hands on the knees as in Gyana Mudra.
- Close the eyes and relax the whole body.
- Draw the tongue outside the mouth and roll it up from the sides to form a channel like a bird's beak.

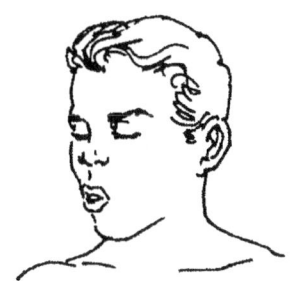

Fig. 7.9: Sheetali Pranayama

- Slowly and deeply inhale the air through it and fill the lungs completely.
- After complete inhalation, withdraw the tongue, close the mouth and exhale through the nose.
- Repeat the exercise 5 to 10 times.
- Gradually increase the rounds upto 15 or even more as well as the duration of each inhalation/exhalation.

Precautions
- This technique should not be practised in a dirty, polluted atmosphere since breathing such air through the mouth transfers it directly into the lungs.
- This pranayama is not suitable for patients suffering from low blood pressure or respiratory disorders, such as asthma and bronchitis.
- People with constipation should also avoid this pranayama.
- Sheetali pranayama should be avoided in winter or in cool climates.

Sheetkari Pranayama
Techniques
- Sit in any comf and relax the whole body.
- Hold the teeth lightly together, keeping the lips open.
- Slightly press the tip of the tongue against the lower front

teeth and then inhale the air. Slowly through the mouth over the tongue with a hissing sound.

- After full inhalation withdraw the tongue and close the mouth and slowly exhale through both nostrils.

- Complete 5 to 10 rounds.

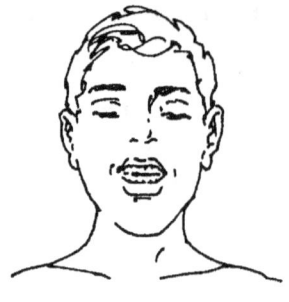

Fig. 7.10: Sheetkari Pranayama

Precautions

As with Sheetali Pranayama. People with infected teeth and gums, missing teeth or dentures should not practise this pranayama.

Meditation

Definition

Patanjali, the original teacher of yoga had described meditation as "the uninterrupted thinking of one thought". Swami Vivekanada had said "Meditation is the focussing of the mind on some object. If the mind acquires concentration on one object it can concentrate on any object whatsoever"

Basic Procedure of Meditation

Through different religions, communities and sects may have some variation in the procedure of meditation, the basic procedure is almost similar in all cases. The main goal in meditation is to withdraw the mind and senses from the surrounding environment and focus the attention on any given object.

Meditation is usually done in the following steps.

Complete Relaxation

Complete relaxation refers to conscious suspension of all movements of the body resulting in relaxation of all skeletal muscles and limpness of the body. Adopting either sitting postures like Padmasana, Sukhasana and Vajrasana or the standing posture.

- Maintain the posture and keep the spine and neck straight

and the whole body relaxed.
- Concentrate your mind on each part of the body one by one starting from the toes to the head.
- Allow each part to relax and feel that it has become relaxed completely.

Awareness of Breathing
- Concentrate completely on the breathing, taking slow, deep and rhythmic breaths.
- Concentrate at the meeting point of both nasal cavities and perceive both the incoming and outgoing breaths.
- Next concentrate on the navel and be fully aware of the contraction and expansion of abdominal muscles during exhalation and inhalation respectively.
- Alternate breathing can also be practised during meditation without causing any wandering thoughts or discomfort.

Awareness of Body Parts
- Concentrate on each part of the body one by one perceiving the sensations and vibrations in each part. Start with the big toe of right foot, moving upwards in the front and back to the head focussing on each part.
- Perceive the body as a whole while assuming or even standing up slowly from the sitting posture.

Awareness of Chakras or Psychic Centres
- While sitting in the relaxed posture, focus the attention on the seven chakras or psychic centres, starting from the Muladhara Chakra or Shakti Kendra.
- Imagine as if the vibrations are flowing from Muladhara Chakra upwards upto Sahasra Chakra or Jyoti Kendra.

| S. | Chakra/Psychic | Location | Corresponding |

No.	Centre		Organ
1.	Muladhara Chakra or Shakti Kendra (centre or energy).	Lower end of spinal cord and genitals.	Gonads- testes/ovaries.
2.	Swadhisthana Chakra or Taijasa Kendra (Centre of bioelectricity).	Below navel and back.	Adrenals, Spleen.
3.	Manipura Chakra.	Above navel and back.	Pancrease and liver.
4.	Anahata Chakra or Ananda Kendra (Centre of bliss).	Chest and heart region.	Thymus.
5.	Vishuddi Chakra/ Kendra (centre of purity).	Throat and back of neck.	Thyroid and parathyroid glands.
6.	Ajna Chakra or Kendra (centre of Intuition.	Darshan centre of eyebrows.	Pituitary gland.
7.	Sahasra Chakra or Jyoti Kendra (centre of enlightenment).	Top of head.	Pineal gland.

Awareness of Psychic Colours

The chakras or psychic centres can be activated by visualizing certain colours which are capable of producing specific vibrations. This is possible by regular practice of meditation.

While perceiving the different chakras or psychic centres, one should visualize particular colour which is specific for it (Refer Table below). This helps in activating these centres and enhancing their physiological functions.

| S.No. | Chakra/Psychic Centre | Colour to be |

		Visualised
1.	Muladhara Chakra of Shakti Kendra.	Red
2.	Swadhisthana Chakra or Taijasa Kendra.	Orange
3.	Manipura Chakra.	Yellow
4.	Anahata Chakra or Ananda Kendra.	Green
5.	Vishuddhi Chakra Kendra.	Blue
6.	Ajna Chakra or Darshan Kendra.	Purple
7.	Sahasra Chakra or Jyoti Kendra.	White

Auto-Suggestion and Resolution

Auto-suggestion refers to repeated recitation of a sentence e.g. "The pain in my knee is disappearing" or "My headache has gone" etc. Auto-suggestion helps in building up faith and belief and the tolerance to bear the disease or its effects. This also brings up physiological changes in the body weakening the forces of disease, mental imbalance and emotional disturbances.

Resolution or contemplation refers to building up healthy and positive attitude towords life. This can be done by repeating. "I will not steal" or "I will tell the truth", or "I will stand first in the class" etc. Repetition of such a resolution helps in overcoming negative attitudes and psychological distortions and develop positive attitudes like truthfulness, amity, fearlessness tolerances, love, sympathy etc.

Role of Meditation in Treatment of Diabetes

- By concentrating on the "Manipura Chakra" which is a psychic centre for pancreas, it is possible to reactivate the sluggish pancreas and increase its function, especially the increase in insulin secretion. This needs regular practice and concentration but results are permanent

- Similarly the "Manipura Chakra" can be activated by visualizing "Yellow" colour which can produce positive vibrations in the pancreas, thereby activating its functional status.

- During the phase of autosuggestion the diabetic person should say repeatedly. "My diabetes is controlled and my blood sugar levels have come down to normal levels." Or "My pancreas is now working perfectly and my diabetes is under conrol." These statements help in bringing about physiological changes in the body and weakening the insensitivity of insulin and increasing its production in the body.

- Regular pratice of meditation stabilizes and strengthens the neuro-muscular, neuro-endocrine and immunological systems keeping the body fit and controlling diabetes.

- Negative thoughts and emotions are controlled helping people to overcome stress which may be one of the precipitating factors of diabetes.

Naturopathy or Nature Cure

Naturopathy or nature cure is the technique of following the rules of nature and exploiting the natural resources like the sun, air, water and soil to cure the various maladies affecting man.

The branch of Naturopathy which are useful for treatment of diabetes are Hydrotherapy, Mud Therapy, and Massage.

Hydrotherapy

Water is very essential for our life. It not only quenches our thirst but also has certain medicinal properties by virtue of its rich mineral content. Water contains copper, carbon, sulphur, phosphorus, iodine, calcium and other valuable minerals and chemicals of medicinal value.

How does hydrotherapy work in treatment of Diabetes?

- Hot water is useful in removing congestion of blood around the pancreas and surrounding organs thereby increasing blood circulation to that area.

- Cold water will reduce swelling and inflammation, and relax the blood vessels in the abdomen, hence normalizing the blood circulation.

- It removes the sluggishness of the pancreas and activates its function of digestion and metabolism.
- Accumulation of toxins and waste products in and around the pancreas is eliminated.

Types of Hydrotherapy Useful for Treatment of Diabetes
Heat Compress
A linen cloth or bandage of about 3 metres length and 30 centimetres width is kept in cold water for a few minutes. After squeezing it dry it is bound around the region of the navel completely. A dry woolen cloth or blanket is wrapped around it to prevent circulation of air and help accumulation of body heat. This has to be left in position for about an hour resulting in perspiration. After removing the compress, the area should be rubbed with a wet cloth and dried with a towel.

Friction Rub
The patient is made to sit with feet immersed in hot water upto the ankle in a tub. The face is washed with cold water. Some ice-cold water is taken in basin and a coarse hand towel is dipped in the water. Each part of the body is rubbed briskly with this towel. After this, the body is covered with a bigger dry towel and rubbed again. This type of bath if taken in the morning is very useful for patients with diabetes.

Alternate Hip Bath or Revulsive Hip Bath
A special type of tub is used in which water covers only the hips and abdomen when the patient sits in it. The tub is filled with water which is filled with hot water between $40^{\circ}C$ to $45^{\circ}C$ and cold water between $10^{\circ}C$ to $20^{\circ}C$. The patient should alternately sit in the hot tub for 5 minutes and in the cold tub for 3 minutes. The head and neck should be kept cold with a cold compress. The treatment should end with a spray of cold water to the hips.

Steam Bath
Steam bath is the most important form of hydrotherapy which eliminates toxins through the skin by inducing sweat. It can be done in a specially designed cabinet or at home. At home a large

bucket may be taken which is big enough to immerse the legs upto the knees in hot water. The temperature of water should be kept moderate. The patient should sit on a stool in an underwear with both legs immersed in water and a cold wet towel on the head. The whole body should be covered upto the neck with a thick blanket. After 15 to 20 minutes, the blanket should be removed and a cold shower taken.

Mud Therapy

Earth provides us with food—our main source of energy. In the same way, earth in the form of mud or clay packs or poultices or even mud baths help in the treatment and prevention of many diseases.

In diabetes the basic defect lies in the lack of metabolism of carbohydrates or sugars which accumulate in the body. Mud therapy helps in activation of the metabolism by stimulating the endocrine and digestive organs. It also helps in the removal of impurities and toxins in the body.

How to Use the Mud

- Use commercially available mud or ordinary white clay. Spread it in the hot sunlight and allow it to dry. If it is very sticky, add some sand to make it fine. Sieve it well and remove stones, dirt and foreign particles. For best results, dissolve mud in water in a container overnight, filter it with a clean cloth and dry the filtrate.
- Always use mud with a clean stick or spatula and never with hands.
- In summer, mud should be dissolved in ice or cold water for better results and in water it should be warm enough.
- For warm mud pack, boil water well and to it add mud.
- Mud which is dissolved in water overnight should be well covered to avoid contamination by dirt, dust, stones and impurities.
- Never re-use the mud which has been used for mud therapy.

Mud Therapy in the Treatment of Diabetes

Mud Pack

Mud or clay is dissolved in preferably warm water till a thick paste is formed. This paste is thickly applied to the abdomen in the area around the navel (without clothes). The average size of mud pack is 1 foot long, 8 inches broad and $1/2$ inch thick which may vary in obese individuals and children.

After applying a mud pack the patient is covered with an old cotton or woolen cloth depending on the weather conditions. The patient should remain in this mud pack for about 30 to 90 minutes, followed by a shower and dried well.

The time of applying mud pack is 2 hours before and 3 to 4 hours after a meal.

Mud Bath

A mud bath may be taken using mud or earth from a place which has been exposed to direct sunlight and open air with no fertilisers used, and adequately hydrated. This mud or earth is mixed with some sand and water and applied to the whole body in the morning. The person should stay in the mild sunshine for about 30 to 40 minutes, applying mud whenever it dries up. At the end a bath is taken with fresh water.

In some centres, a special tub is designed which allows people to lie in it covered upto the chin in mud. This allows them to lie comfortably in the tub for about 30 minutes, followed by a bath.

Massage

Massage is an excellent form of passive exercise as well as cure for many ailments. It is an integral part of Naturopathy as well as Ayurveda.

It tones up the nervous system activating each and every part of the brain. It accelerates the elimination of toxins and waste materials from the body through the lungs, kidneys, bowels and skin. It also boosts up the blood circulation, digestion and metabolism.

Massage useful for treatment of diabetes
- Kneading
- Clapping
- Pounding
- Vibrations

Kneading

Kneading is a very important technique of massage used for treatment of diabetes. Using both hands deep pressure is exerted on the abdomen especially in the region around the navel. This is done for 10-15 minutes preferably empty stomach in the morning.

This produces an increased flow of blood to pancreas and other organs enhancing the process of digestion and absorption of nutrients. Regular massage can even stimulate the sluggish islet cells of the pancreas and increase their metabolic activity.

Clapping

This is a heavy movement used on the liver and pancreas. The patient is made to lie supine in such a way that the operator faces him from the right side. The upper abdomen is covered with a blanket. The operator (naturopath) strikes the abdomen with the inner aspect of right hand, with fingers loosely clenched and force transmitted from the shoulder.

The technique of clapping produces a mechanical stimulation of islet cells of pancreas whereby secretion of insulin is stimulated and its activity enhanced.

Pounding

This is similar to clapping except for the part that both the hands are used alternately on the abdomen and the force used is slightly heavier.

This technique should be done only by an experienced naturopath.

Vibrations

Using one or both hands vibrations are performed on the abdomen. The movement is of fine shaking of abdomen by slight movements of the fingers or wrists. These movements have a soothing effect on the abdomen, stimulating the digestive juices and hormone secretion.

Coarse vibrations can be done by keeping one hand on the back (spine) and the other on the abdomen and moving the two hands with the breath held in expiration.

Medicated oils

For treatment of diabetes, massage with certain oils gives excellent results. The oils community used are cottonseed oil, sesame (til) oil, castor oil, mustard oil, olive oil and cocunut oil. For better results these oils are combined with eucalyptus, comphor, musk or myrrh.

Jojoba oil along with essential oils such as cedar, pine musk, cinnamon, juniper, basel, ginger, cumin, cayenne, clove yarrow, grapeseed, avocado and canola give very good results in diabetic patients.

These oils are usually warmed and applied on the abdomen especially around the navel for 15 to 20 minutes on an empty stomach followed by a warm water bath.

Medical Treatment (Allopathic)

There are four types of medical treatment and the patient may shift from one group to the other temporarily or permanently depending on the severity of disease, response to treatment and special situations.

The four types of treatment are as follows:
1. Diet alone.
2. Diet + (Oral) tablets.
3. Diet + insulin injections.
4. Diet + insulin + tablets.

Different Types of Diabetics and Treatment

Types of diabetic	Types of treatment
1. Young diabetic (< 40 years).	Diet
2. Middle aged and elderly (Obese) (> 40 years).	Diet alone or Diet + tablets or Diet + insulin.
3. Middle-aged and elderly. (non-obese) (> 40 years)	Diet + tablets or Diet + insulin.
4. Pregnant diabetics.	Diet + insulin.
5. During ketosis, operations, infections, uncontrolled diabetes.	Diet + insulin.

Those patients of diabetes, who do not improve after modification in their diet is made, have to be supplemented with medicines.

The improvement has to be gauged in 2 ways:
- Decrease in their body weight.
- Decrease in the level of blood sugar.

The two types of medicines which are commonly used are:
- Oral medicines in the form of tablets or capsules.
- Insulin injections.

Oral Medicines

Different types of patients with different stages of disease may require one or more types of tablets and/or insulin injections. There are various factors, which determine whether one patient will benefit from one or more types of medicines. The family physician or diabetologist who is treating the patient determines this. Normally the patients who are prescribed or who may benefit from oral medicines are given below:

Types of Diabetics who are Prescribed Tablets

- Middle-aged and elderly individuals with type II Diabetes.
- Individuals who have been diagnosed to have diabetes of less than 5 years duration.
- Patients who have failed with dietary treatment and exercise.
- Patients who have lost weight with dietary treatment and exercise but blood sugar is not reduced.
- Patients who cannot be prescribed injections because of irregular meals and life-style.
- Patients with mild diabetes who have visual difficulty and cannot use insulin injections.
- Those who regularly develop very low levels of blood sugar with insulin.
- Those who show no fall in blood sugar with insulin (insulin resistance).
- Those who cannot afford the cost of insulin injections.

- Patients who are reluctant to use injections as a form of treatment.

Salient Features of Oral Medicines (Tablets)

	Generic Name	Brand	Dose (mg/day)	Frequency	Common Side Effects
1.	Glipizide	Glynase	2.5 to 40	1 to 3 times	Vomiting, abdominal pain, loose stools.
2.	Chlorpropamide	Diabenese	100 to 500	once a day	Skin rashes, liver disorder.
3.	Glibenclamide	Daonil	2.5 to 15	1 to 2 times	Reaction with alcohol.
4.	Gliclazide	Diamicron	80 to 320	twice daily	Weight gain.
5.	Tolbutamide	Rastinon	500 to 3000	2 to 3 times	Reduced blood sodium.
6.	Phenformin	DBI	25 to 100	1 to 4 times	Vomiting, reduced appetite, taste.
7.	Metformin	Glyciphage	500 to 3000	2 to 3 times	Change, loose stools, muscle weakness, Vitamin B12 not absorbed, increased blood, lactic acid.
8.	Glimepiride	Amaryl	1 to 6	1 to 2 times	Liver dysfunction, rashes.
9.	Repaglinide	Rapilin	0.5 to 16	Before each meal	Vomiting, loose stools, visual problem, rashes.
10.	Pioglitazone	Pioglit	15 to 30	once daily	Weight gain, headache swelling of body, visual disturbances, joint pain, impotence.
11.	Rosiglitazone	Result	4 to 8	1 to 2 times	Weight gain, vomiting, loose stools, headache, swelling of body.

Points to Remember

- Beneficial effect of these medicines is usually seen within 3 to 4 weeks of treatment.
- Those patients who do not benefit from one group of tablets, another group may be added by the doctor.
- Certain medicines are known to interfere with the blood sugar lowering action of these tablets. So the patient should always consult a doctor even for simple painkillers.
- Proper spacing of meals is important and prolonged fasting is to be avoided to prevent sudden fall in blood sugar levels.
- Regular blood and urine tests are required to monitor the effect of these medicines.
- Never take alcoholic drinks when on oral medicines especially the sulphonylureas.
- Patients on these medicines, who become pregnant or develop severe infection have to get operated, should contact their doctor immediately because they have to be prescribed insulin injections instead of tablets in such cases.
- Tablets should always be taken, immediately before or during a meal or else blood sugar level may suddenly drop down.

Insulin Injections

In certain individuals with diabetes who have very minimal production of insulin in the pancreas those who do not benefit from treatment with dietary modification and tablets, insulin injections may be prescribed. A list of the type of diabetic patients who are normally prescribed insulin injections or those who may benefit from them is given below:

- Young individuals with type 1 diabetes.
- Patients with diabetes of more than 15 years duration.
- Patients with keto-acidosis or coma.
- Patients with diabetes during pregnancy.
- Diabetics who have to undergo major operations.

- Diabetics with associated infection, diarrhoea and vomiting, during an accident and heart attack and those with nerve damage.
- Patients with liver disease or sulpha allergy or pancreatic disease where oral tablets are not to be given.
- Patients whose blood sugar is not lowered in spite of dietary treatment.

Types of Insulin

According to the source insulins are bovine – which is derived from pancreas of cattle, porcine—derived from pancreas of pigs and human produced by recombinant DNA.

According to duration of action insulin are short-acting, intermediate-acting and long-acting.

According to strength of injection:
- Insulin injections are available in the strengths of 20, 40, 80 and 100 Iu/ml. Human insulin is absorbed faster than porcine and latter faster than bovine. Zinc and protamine when added to insulin delays its release from site of injection and prolongs effect of insulin.

Different types of insulin and their salient features are given in the table below:

Different Types of Insulin and their Activity

Type of Insulin	Onset of Action (Minutes)	Peak (Hours)	Duration (Hours)
Short-acting			
1. Regular or Plain	15-30	2-5	6-8
2. Insulin Zinc (Semilentre)	30-60	6-10	12-16
Intermediate-acting			
1. Isophane (NPH)	1-2	4-12	18-22
2. Insulin Zinc (lente)	1-3	7-15	18-22
Long-acting			
1. Insulin Zinc (ultralente)	3-4	6-16	24-28
2. Protamine Zinc Insulin	3-4	10-15	24-36

Storage of Injections

Insulin injections should be stored in the refrigerator at 40°F. Direct exposure to sunlight may reduce its activity.

Where to Inject?

Insulin injection may be given in the outer aspect of the arms, anterior part of forearms, anterior part of abdomen below the waist, front of the thighs above the knees, and, upper part of buttocks. The site of injection should be changed every time so that at one site injection is given after every 15-20 days.

How to Inject?

Step 1: Take out the vial containing insulin from the refrigerator and load (fill) the insulin syringe upto the required mark.

Step 2: Clean the site where injection is to be given with spirit or Savlon or Dettol using a cotton swab and allow it to dry.

Step 3: Lift up the skin and fat of the selected site between thumb and forefinger of left hand.

Step 4: Insert the needle through the selected site at an angle of 45 degrees using your right hand.

Step 5: Pull out the plunger slightly to ensure that the needle is not in a blood vessel.

Step 6: Slowly push the plunger inside the syringe and push the medicine through the skin and fat.

Step 7: Remove the needle and syringe and massage slightly with cotton swab.

Complications of Insulin Injections

Sometimes a few side effects may be seen with the usage of insulin injections. They are as follows:

- Low blood sugar levels may be observed suddenly especially if the patient is not taking meals at proper time or in sufficient quantity.

- High blood sugar levels may be suddenly seen in a few patients who have been well-controlled with some dose of insulin.
- Swelling of the feet may be seen temporarily on starting the injections for the first time.
- Some patients may develop resistance to insulin either temporarily during keto-acidosis, infections etc. or permanently with no fall of sugar levels inspite of high doses.
- Itching, and skin rashes at the site of injection may be seen in a few individuals.
- Loss of fat at the site of injection and surrounding areas may be seen.
- Blurring of vision before starting treatment may become worse in some cases.
- Some patients report increase in appetite and weight after starting injections.

Points to Remember

- All diabetics except very old, bedridden, blind, mentally retarded or those with unsteady hand should learn to inject themselves. This makes them independent and ensures uninterruped treatment.
- Injections should be given a few minutes before meals.
- Injections should never be given near scar tissue where absorption is slow.
- In infections like common cold, fever, boils etc higher dose may be required.
- Patients with kidney disorders may have a prolonged action of insulin.
- Initially blood sugar level may have to be checked about 4 times a day i.e. before meals and at bed time until an optimum dose is calculated.

- During an emotional distress, the dosage of insulin may have to be increased.

- In athletes thighs and arms may not be used for injecting insulin since in such individuals exercise of these areas cause rapid absorption of insulin.

A comparative study of treatment with tablets and insulin injections is outlined below:

Comparison of Treatment with Tablets and Insulin Injections

Treatment with Tablets	Treatment with Insulin Injections
1. More readily acceptable by patient.	Sometimes unacceptable.
2. Patient can treat himself independently.	Medical supervision is required especially in the initial phase of treatment.
3. Can be taken easily.	Injections are painful and require care and caution.
4. No resistance to medicines is seen.	Resistance is common.
5. Action of medicines is mainly on the liver.	Action is mainly on the muscles and tissues.
6. Low blood sugar less frequent and less severe.	More frequent and more severe.
7. No local reactions.	Local reactions at site of injection.
8. Drug-interaction common.	Drug interaction rare
9. Toxic reactions and severe side effects may occur.	Very rarely seen.
10. Dosage not flexible.	Dosage is flexible.
11. Not useful during pregnancy	Very useful in pregnancy
12. Not useful for type 1 Diabetes.	Very useful for type 1 diabetes
13. Cannot be used in those with liver or kidney disorder.	Can be used.
14. Not very useful in infections, operations etc.	Very useful in such cases.
15. Not useful for malnourished patients.	Can be used in malnourished patients.
16. Not used in severe, uncontrolled disease.	Very useful in severe, uncontrolled disease.
17. Long term effects on liver and heart common.	Not usually seen.

Ayurvedic Treatment of Diabetes

Treatment of diabetes in Ayurveda is not just confined to medicines, diet and exercise but other measures are also involved. This difference in the approach to the disease is due to the difference in the concept of the disease. In Ayurveda it is believed that any disease is due to imbalance in the doshas i.e. one or more doshas may increase or decrease. Diabetes is commonly believed to be due to increase in VATA-DOSHA. In some individuals depending on their inherent nature there may be an increase in PITTA or KAPHA DOSHAS. Thus the principle of treatment in Ayurveda is to bring about a balance in the three DOSHAS.

The methods of treatment may be divided into three groups: Preliminary treatment, specific treatment and dietary modification.

I. Preliminary Treatment

The preliminary treatment is aimed at bringing about a balance in the doshas. The preliminary treatment varies according to the state of nutrition of the patient i.e. whether the person is obese and overnourished or malnourished.

The obese diabetics are given preliminary treatment as follows:

Shehana or Drinking of Oily Substances

Patients on first visit to a Ayurvedacharya are asked to drink oils like mustard oil, neem oil as preliminary treatment. This is given depending on the digestive powers of the individual. Those with mild digestive powers are asked to use oil for one day only while those with moderate digestion for 2-3 days and those with strong digestion for 5-7 days. Charaka-Samhita, the Bible of Ayurveda, claims that this measure removes the Vata Dosha from the body.

Vamana or Induced Vomiting

Certain medicines are given to induce vomiting in obese diabetics. This is done to remove the kapha dosha from the body. This is also one of the five measures for purification of the body known as panchakarma.

Virechana or Induced Diarrhoea

Certain medicines are given to induce purgation or diarrhoea to remove the pitta doshas from the body and also to purify the body.

Samsarjana or Dietary Regulation

Obese individuals are then started on light diet consisting of semi-sold diet like boild rice, gruel, daliya and gradually put on cereal diet consisting of less of fat and carbohydrates.

All these measures are done only under the supervision of a Ayurvedic physician.

The basic objective of treatment in malnourished diabetics is to destroy the doshas, which are present in the body of the individual. This consists of following measures:

Sanshaman or Destruction of Unbalanced Doshas

This is mainly done by asking the diabetic individual to eat or drink the following substances:

- Barley boiled in water.
- Soup of non-vegetarian origin e.g. chicken, pigeon.
- Watery dals e.g. moong dal.
- Soups made by boiling bitter gourd (Karela).
- Soup made by boiling jambu fruit (Jamun).
- Haldi (Turmeric), deodhar, trifla, nagarmotha in equal quantities powdered and decoction made.
- Juice of amla and Haldi churan.
- Medicated ghee e.g. Shalmali Grith.

Nourishing Diet

A protein rich, easily digestible diet with least content of fat and carbohydrates.

Medicines to Increase Appetite and Nutrition

Certain medicines like Devdarurishta and Chandan Asava are known to improve the appetite and nutritional status of the individual.

II. Specific Treatment

This is directed at bringing about a control in the disease by applying certain meaures externally or internally to the body.

a) External Treatment

Massage with medicated oils: Many diabetics benefit by massaging their body daily with medicated oils containing trifla, daruhaldi, barley, amla, or patent oils like Mehmihir Tel, Prameha Mihir Tel. The massage is followed by a shower bath.

Body pack: The patient is asked to apply a thick layer or pack after grinding khas, dalchini, elaichi (small), agroo and sandal and making a paste applied to the whole body.

Sunbath: A sunbath early in the morning is very nourishing for the body.

Swimming, horse riding: Exercises in the form of swimming or horse riding are very useful.

Yogasanas: Certain Yogasanas are found to be very useful for controlling diabetes especially in the early part of the disease. These asanas are advised to be done before sunrise after emptying the bowel and bladder and preferably to be done daily for about 30-60 minutes. The important asanas are Sarvangasana, Paschimottanasana, Dhanurasana, Mayurasana, Bhujangasana, Uddiyanbandh and Nouli Kriya.

b) Internal Treatment

Internal treatment is done using Ayurvedic medicines in the form of tablets (Vati, Ras), Churan, Bhasma (heavy metal powder); liquid (Asavas, Arista); Ark (tincture), decoctions), Avleh (paste) and medicated oils (tels).

According to Charak-Samhita, the following medicines have been used in the treatment of diabetes:

- Vasanta Kusumakara Ras 0.5 to 1 gm given with haridra-amalaki churan twice daily was observed to improve the function of the pancreas and improve general debility and weakness.

- Brahath Vangeshwar Ras 125mg -240mg along with decoction of Vijayasar reduces blood sugar levels.
- Indravati 1 to 2 tablets daily are very useful
- Chandraprabha Vati 2 - 4 tablets twice daily with milk.
- Shatavar Ras with equal quantities of milk
- Mehkalanal Ras 240 mg every morning with milk.
- Hemanath Ras 200-250 mg twice or thrice daily.
- Vasanta Tilaka Ras 200-250 mg twice or thrice daily.
- Saptarangyadi Vati 1 to 2 tablets twice or thrice daily.
- Mehmudkar Vati 1 tablet once or twice daily.
- Vedvidya Vati 1 tablet once or twice daily with juice of amla.
- Mehkesri Ras 1 tab once daily with milk and rice.
- Sarveshwar Ras 1 tab once daily.
- Shilajit in the pure form of Shilajitwadi Vati 250-500mg daily in divided doses. It is a wonder drug, which is believed to remove all the doshas and cure diabetes in early stages.
- Swarnmakshik Bhasm 120-250 mg twice daily.

The medicinal plants or extracts found to be useful for the treating of diabetes are as follows:

- Soft portion of the seeds of Jamun powdered and 15 to 45 gm swallowed with water twice or thrice daily or 60mg of fruit and seeds of Jamun boiled with 300ml of water for 30 minutes. Then grind and filter the portion and divide into 3 parts, each taken once daily. This is a very good remedy for reducing blood sugar.
- Juice of fruits and leaves of Bitter gourd (Karela) 25 to 100 gm once or twice daily preferably on an empty stomach.
- Bimbi (Trikol) leaves ground into a powdered form and taken 3-6gm twice daily with water or 15ml of juice taken twice daily.

- Kaith (Wood apple) plant taken in the form of powdered churan 3mg or tincture 15ml once or twice daily.

- Soft portion of the seeds and flowers of Katakkaranj taken orally as churan or applied as paste on skin diseases due to diabetes.

- Leaves made into a paste (1 gm) of Udumbar (Goolar) tree or fruit juice (15ml) or soft portion of root (1 gm) given once or twice daily.

- Other useful plants which can be given as a whole in the form of churan, decoction or juice are Tuvrak, Sitaphal, Haridki, Amla, Guduchi, Kushta, Neem leaves, flowers and stem, fruits and leaves of Drumstick, Patola, Bilva.

Patent medicines consisting of combination of above medicines:

JK - 22	Hyponidd
jumbolin	Glucomap
Diabecon	
Madhumehari	Madhumeharyog

Ayurvedic Treatment of Complications

The best treatment of complications is to control the disease and hence prevent onset of complications of diabetes.

Kidney Diseases and High Blood Pressure

Certain Ayurvedic medicines are useful for treating the above complications. They are Juice of the root of white punarva plant, Shweta parpati, Punarnava mandoor, Chandra prabha vati, and soft part of seeds of Kata Karanj.

Nerve Diseases

Medicines for treatment of nerve diseases are powder of Jyotishmati, powder of Neeli, Juice of neem leaves or palash, sapta parnimol and pure shilajit + sharpunka root each 10gm mixed together and made into tablets of 250mg with 1 to 2 tablets twice or thrice daily with Trifla decoction.

Diabetic Coma
This is managed as follows:

- Immediate treatment is to apply nausadar + lime + camphor in the form of snuff intra-nasal to bring the patient to consciousness.

- Bel and neem leaves in the form of juice in equal portions applied on the forehead and head, the technique known as Shirodhara.

- Body application of Hemanashu Oil and 1000 times washed ghee.

- Oral medicines like Murchantak Ras, Yogender Ras, Chandarakant Ras, Brahat Kasturi, Bhairav Ras, Dashmool decoction or arishta (liquid), Guggul, Bala, Rasna.

Heart Disease
- Haritki Churan + churan of neem leaves + garlic (without skin) in equal amounts with 15ml of tincture of Palash 4 times a day.

- Leaves of Vasa and stem of Giloy made into a juice and 25 ml taken twice daily.

- Regular usage of about 100mg of garlic and onion is believed to reduce cholesterol content of blood.

Eye Complications
- Clean eyes with decoction of Trifla.

- Swallow Trifla churan + root of white Punarava with water.

Gangrene
- Washing of feet with decoction of neem followed by neem oil application regularly.

- Local application of any one of the oils—Juice of leaves of neem and sharpunkha, Punarnavadi paste and oil Trifla paste Jatyadi Tel (oil), Prameha Mihir Tel.

- For oral usage tincture of Palash mixed with juice of palash plant and neem juice.

Carbuncle
- Local application of neem leaves paste or Katakaranj flowers and soft portions of seeds as paste.
- Oral usage of either Shrestadi Vati 1-2 tablets twice or thrice daily or Kutaki and Chirayata powder dissolved in water and filtered and solution taken twice daily.

III. Dietary Modification

Diabetics who are obese should have a low calorie, fat free diet while malnourished diabetics should have protein rich, medium calorie and fat-free diet. Due to the concept of vata, pitta and kapha certain food substances have to be avoided since they are known to increase one or more of these doshas. The food substances, which can be given freely, are as follows:

- **Cereals:** Unpolished rice, barley, all dals.
- **Vegetables:** Tinda, red pumpkin (Kaddu), green leafy vegetables, peas, tomato, turnip leaves, radish leaves, bottle gourd (ghia), sponge gourd (turai), parval.
- **Fruits:** Jamun, orange, apple, and pomegranate.
- **Meat:** Pigeon, rabbit, deer, duck, parrot, chicken.

Food Substances to be Avoided
- **Cereals:** Polished rice, wheat, jowar, moong, urad, masoor, chana, lobia.
- **Vegetables:** Carrot, beetroot, potato, sweet potato, turnip, radish, cauliflower.
- **Fruits:** Grapes, mango, water-melon, pear etc.
- Dry fruits and nuts.
- Oils and ghee.
- Full cream milk and its products.

- Sweets of any kind.
- Syrups, juices.
- Alcohol, vinegar.

Home Remedies for Treatment of Diabetes

- Take 10gm of fenugreek (Methi) seeds and 10gm of dried bitter gourd (Karela) and powder it well. Take 1 teaspoonful of this powder empty stomach with water daily.
- Take a few raw bananas, cut them into pieces and dry them. Grind them into a fine powder and take 1 teaspoonful of this powder with pure cow's milk daily.
- Take 1 cup of carrot juice and $1/2$ cup of palak jiuce and add $1/2$ teaspoonful of powdered jeera (cumin seed) and a pinch of salt and drink it daily.
- Drink juice of a medium-sized radish daily after lunch.
- Early in the morning chew four to five tender neem leaves daily.
- Chew 4 to 5 leaves of Jamun (Black Plum) along with a pinch of rock salt early in the morning.
- Take a branch of gulmohar tree and dip it in about 1 litre of water. Drink one cup of this water twice daily until it lasts.
- Take 100gm of seeds of Jamun (black plum) and 4 to 5 dried amla (Indian gooseberry) and powder them. Take 1 teaspoon of thus powder daily on empty stomach with water.
- Take the roots of Bael tree, dry them and powder them. Take 1 teaspoonful of this powder with $1/2$ teaspoonful of juice of bael leaves.
- Take 20gm of papaya, 5gm catechu (Katha) 1 supari cut into pieces and boil in $1/2$ litre of water till a decoction is prepared. Drink this daily after meals.

Magnetotherapy

Definition

Magnetotherapy is a branch of medicine in which human diseases are treated by the application of magnets to the body of the patients. It is the simplest, cheapest and painless system of medicine with absolutely no side-effects.

Treatment of Diabetes by Magnetotherapy

Diabetes can be effectively controlled and even cured by using magnetotherapy in the following ways :

- The traditional treatment of diabetes is to keep the North Pole of the high-power cast alloy magnet under the palm of the right hand and the South Pole under the palm of the left hand for 10 minutes twice daily.

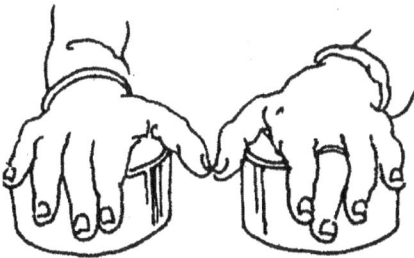

Fig. 7.11: North Pole under right palm and South Pole under left palm

- If this method does not effectively control blood sugar levels in 2-3 weeks, the North Pole of the above magnet should be directly placed on the pancreas and South pole on the back just opposite to North Pole. This should be done for 5-10 minutes twice a day.

- In case of uncontrolled and chronic diabetes, electromagnets can be applied along with the high-power magnets at the level of pancreas for 5-10 minutes daily.

- Specially designed belly (abdominal) belt can be useful for patients with recently diagnosed diabetes. This belt is designed to cover the abdomen and back with magnets which are in contact with the pancreas. This belt can be used for 30 to 60 minutes twice daily.

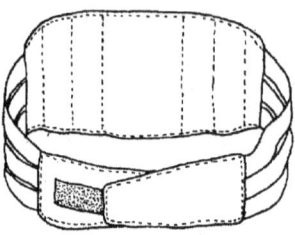
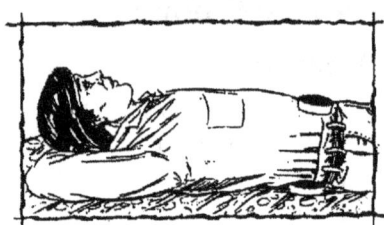

Fig. 7.12 (a): Belly Belt   *Fig. 7.12 (b): North Pole on Pancreas & South Pole on Back*

- Water magnetised with North and South Pole can be taken simultaneously in the dose of 2 to 3 ounces 3 to 4 times daily for adults and in smaller doses for children daily. This helps in boosting up the digestive and metabolic systems of the body.

Adverse Effects

These are very rarely seen, especially in those using high power of electro magnets. The effects reported are as follows:

Mild tingling sensation in the hands and feet, a feeling of warmth in the body, heaviness of head, dryness of tongue, increased urge for urination, mild giddiness, and sweating in the areas on contact with magnets.

Precautions

- The ideal time for using magnetotherapy is in the morning, preferably empty stomach and after a bath.
- Avoid eating or drinking cold things for at least one hour after applying high power magnets.
- Since magnetotherapy produces some heat in the body, bath should not be taken for at least one hour after treatment.
- If high power or medium power magnets are applied after full meals they may cause nausea.
- High power magnets should not be applied to pregnant women, very weak ladies and to children.

- High power magnets should not be applied directly to delicate organs of the body namely eyes, head and heart.
- Watches should not be allowed to come in contact with magnets unless they are anti-magnetic or magnet-proof.
- When high power magnets are applied for long periods they may produce heaviness in head, giddiness, yawning, tingling in nerves etc. Discontinue contact with magnets and rest immediately.
- Opposite poles of high power magnets should not be brought near each other face to face as they attract each other with great force.
- When high power or medium power magnets are not in use they should be kept joined with a keeper so that their magnetism is not wasted and they are not demagnetised soon.
- When taking magnetic treatment under palms, it is not necessary to remove gold or silver rings from the finger.
- While using high-power magnets, one should sit on the wooden stool or chair and also keep a plank under the feet.

Acupressure and Reflexology

It is believed that in our body there is presence of bioenergy or bioelectrical activity which makes us move, breathe, eat and even think. This energy is "called "Prana" or ""chetana" in India while Chinese call it "chi" which consists of "Ÿin" or negative force and "Ÿang" or positive force. These forces or bioenergy flow through definite channels in the body called meridians or "Jing".

There are 14 meridians in our body of which 12 are located in pairs on either side of the body while the remaining two are single and lie each on the front and back of the body. The 12 paired meridians comprise 6 "Ÿin" meridians starting from the toes or mid-part of the body and reaching the head or fingers and 6 "Ÿang" meridians in the reverse direction.

These meridians maintain the flow of bioelectricity and are connected with the main organs or systems of the body. One end of each meridian lies in the hand, the leg or the face and the other in the main organ after which it is named. This is the reason why pressure applied to a particular point on the hand or the leg affects the remote organ connected with this point.

The 14 meridians are large intestine meridian, stomach meridian, small intestine meridian, bladder meridian, triple warmer meridian, gall bladder meridian, lung meridian, spleen meridian, kidney meridian, heart meridian, heart constrictor or pericardium meridian, liver meridian, governing vessel meridian and conception vessel meridian.

Each of the 14 main meridians has subsidiary meridians. If the flow of bioenergy in a meridian is not proper, it can be corrected by stimulating certain points on the meridian by applying pressure on them. Thus the disease of that organ can be eliminated and the pain in these points is relieved as soon as the disease is eliminated.

Pain on any point on the body is possibly a symptom of some disorder in an organ or in a system of the body. If pressure is methodically applied on this point, the disease or disorder can be alleviated.

Effects of Acupressure

- It reduces pain of different types e.g. joint pain, headache, backache, toothache, sprains etc.

- It also has a tranquilising or sedative effect on the brain. If an EEG is done while doing acupressure it shows depression of delta & theta waves.

- It strengthens the body's natural resistance power due to which the respiratory rate, heart beat, blood pressure, body temperature and metabolism become normal. There is also increase in the red and white blood cells and gamma globulins and cholesterol and triglycerides are decreased.

- Depression , anxiety , stress and tension are controlled with acupressure due to its effect on the brain.

- Muscles and joints are strengthened by acupressure and are useful in treatment of polio, paralysis and other neuromuscular disorders.

Advantages of Acupressure

- It is an easy, simple, effective form of treatment.
- It can be done in the privacy of one's home.
- Treatment can be done as frequently as possible.
- No money is required to be spent to get benefits of treatment.
- No side-effects are seen with this treatment.
- In this form of treatment the person looks after his own health.
- In some cases acupressure can be used as a first aid measure till the doctor arrives or if the patient is admitted to the hospital.
- It helps prevent relapses of the diseases.
- If associates with other forms of treatment gives a speedy relief.
- It increases the efficiency of organs & systems of body & strengthens joints and muscles.
- Even in serious diseases it prevents aggravation of symptoms.
- It establishes the convention of touch communication or touch healing and establishes rapport between doctor & patient.

Reflexology or Zone Therapy

Reflexology refers to the form of treatment which involves giving massage to certain reflex areas of the feet and hands.

The body is divided into 10 longitudinal zones. If a straight line is drawn through the centre of the body, the whole body may be divided into five zones on either side of the body. Zone one extends from the thumb, up the arm to the brain and then down to the big toe, zone two extends from second finger, up the arm to the brain and down to the third toe. Similarly, the other zones of equal width occur through the body from front to back. They are like segments of the body & not fine lines like acupuncture meridian lines. The line marking between each zone extends from the web of finger to the web of the toe. Whichever parts of the body are found within a certain zone, these parts will be linked to one another by energy flow within the zone and can therefore affect one another. Treatment is done by applying pressure to accessible areas within the same zone. Pressure is applied using clothes pegs, metal combs, elastic bands & metal probes around the hands and fingers as well as toes, ankles, wrists, elbows or knees. The amount of pressure applied should be between 2 and 20 lbs for an interval of 30 seconds to 5 minutes.

The reflex areas of the feet and hands are divided into transverse zones. Zone one refers to all parts of the body above the shoulder girdle, zone two refers to those parts between the shoulder girdle and wrist. Zone three refers to organs below the waist.

Technique of Reflexology

The thumb is held bent and the side and end of the thumb is pressed into the part of the foot or hand to be treated. The other fingers of the hand will rest gently around the foot. Certain meridians are present in the soles of feet and their massage in the direction of flow of energy, stimulates the organ. Massaging in the opposite direction gives a soothing effect.

Acupressure points useful in treatment of Diabetes

Certain acupressure points when pressed are likely to result in reduction of blood sugar levels. These are as follows:

- Acupressure points in the centre of the palm in alignment with the bottom of the ring finger.
- Acupressure points on the soles of the feet, one third from the base of the toe next to the big toe and two-thirds above the heel.
- About 2" below the outer side of knee cap. (ST 36)
- About 2" above the elbow joint. (LI 11)

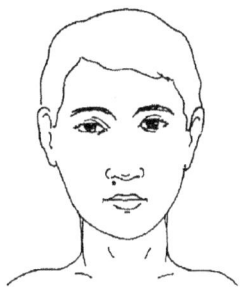

Fig. 7.13: Acupressure point on the upper lip

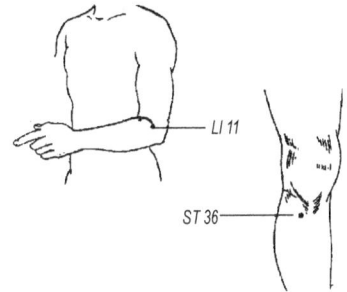

Fig. 7.14: Acupressure points on the knee & elbow

- Acupressure point on the upper lip just near the entrance to right nostril.
- Two points each about $2\frac{1}{2}$" below and $1\frac{1}{2}$" on either side of spine knob on the neck between the second and third vertebrae. (Point No. 194)
- Two points on either side of spine at the level of 11th and 12th thoracic vertebrae. (Point No. 200)
- Two points on either side of spine at the level of 2nd and 3rd lumbar vertebrae. (Point No. 203)
- The acupressure point on the ear as shown in the figure.

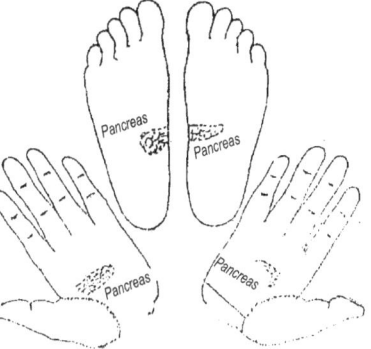

Fig. 7.15: Reflex areas in the palms & soles

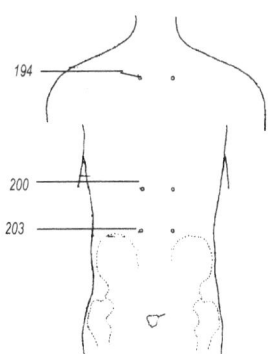

Fig. 7.16: Acupressure point on the back

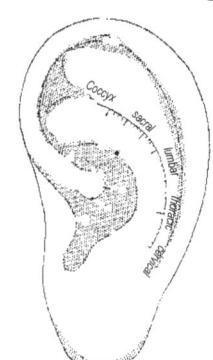

Fig. 7.17: Acupressure point on the ear

Colour Therapy

Colour therapy or Chromotherapy refers to treatment of diseases using different colours. This is usually done in the following manner:

- Direct radiation to the affected part / organ of the body.
- Application of oils, ghee, glycerine etc. charged with specific colour to the affected part.
- Drinking water irradiated in specific coloured bottles.
- Using medicines charged with specific colours.
- Eating specific coloured food items.
- Inhaling gases charged in coloured containers.
- Wearing clothes of specific colours.
- Living/sleeping in a room painted with the specific colours.

How it Works?

Colour is a form of energy which produces certain physiological changes in the body which help in controlling the disease and keeping the body fit.

Yellow is the colour of the pancreas. It is a mixture of red and green rays. The red colour has a stimulating effect while the green vibrations help in the repair of the disease process. Hence it is very beneficial for the treatment of diabetes.

It acts in the following ways:

- It helps in the stimulation of flow of the insulin from the islet cells of the pancreas.
- It increases the digestion of food substances including the carbohydrates by enhancing the function of digestive enzymes.
- It removes toxins from the body and the blood.
- It activates the lymphatic and urinary systems.
- It activates the mood and removes depression.
- It controls the blood sugar and prevents the deterioration in the function of pancreas and delays onset of complications.

Use of Colour Therapy in the Treatment of Diabetes

Direct Radiation: Take a little lamp and attach it with a yellow coloured bulb or cover the existing bulb with yellow-coloured cellophane paper. Apply the direct rays of light from this lamp to the abdomen especially in the region of the pancreas for about 10-15 minutes daily.

Early morning sunbath on the exposed abdomen for 15-20 minutes can also give good results.

Local Application of Irradiated Oil, Ghee

Take a yellow coloured bottle or a white coloured bottle covered with yellow cellophane paper. Fill it with coconut oil, mustard oil, olive oil or ghee and place it on a dry wooden board exposed to direct sunlight for 45 days. It should be kept in the sunlight during the day and in a safe place at night. In case of cloudy/rainy days, artificial light may be used.

This irradiated oil can be used to massage the abdomen, especially the pancreatic region.

Drinking Irradiated Water

Using the procedure given above, water can be charged in yellow-coloured bottles. This should be drunk in the dose of 1 cup early in the morning and ½ cup before lunch and dinner.

Inhaling Yellow Coloured "Air"

An empty yellow-coloured bottle can be kept in the sunlight for about an hour. After removing the cork, the sun-charged "air" in the bottle should be inhaled for a few minutes. This should be repeated thrice daily. This therapy can also improve the function of the pancreas.

Eating Specific Coloured Food Items

Consuming fruits and vegetables which are yellow or orange in colour can also help in the treatment of Diabetes. Examples of such fruits and vegetables are carrots, oranges, apricots, peaches, red berries, water-melon, beet root, radish, red cabbage and red spinach.

Music Therapy

Definition of Music Therapy

Music Therapy is a form of treatment using music and musical instruments in order to restore, maintain and improve physical, physiological, psychological and spiritual health and well-being.

Benefits of Music Therapy

Music therapy when used brings about following benefits or changes in patients and individuals:

- It produces reduction in anxiety and stress often producing sedation and even sleep.
- It can alleviate pain and discomfort in conjunction with anesthesia or pain medication.
- It can bring about positive changes in mood and emotional states.
- It can counteract apprehension or fear.
- It can lessen muscle tension bringing about relaxation of the body.
- Music therapy brings about active participation of the patient in his treatment.
- The length of stay in the hospital or treatment period is decreased.
- An emotional bond develops between the patient, his family members and the doctors.
- This type of therapy is enjoyed by all.
- The whole period of therapy forms a meaningful time spent together in a positive and creative way.
- It improves communication skills and physical coordination in spastic and mentally retarded patients.

Medical Application of Music Therapy

Music therapy has been found to be useful in the treatment of the following diseases:

Sleep disorders, behavioural disorders in children, mental retardation, stammering and speech disorders, psychiatric illnesses - anxiety neurosis, depression, schizophrenia, dementia and alzheimer's disease, arthritis, stroke, acute and chronic pain, hypertension, polio, tinnitus, epilepsy, polio, drug addiction and head injury.

How Music Therapy Helps Patients of Diabetes

- It increases the digestive and metabolic activity in the body—increasing the secretions of digestive enzymes and hormones including insulin.

- It stabilizes the blood pressure and heart rate and hence prevents complications of the heart.

    There is improvement in the cardiac output or blood circulation which invigorates the whole body.

- Active participation in music and dance enhances activity of nerves and muscles and prevents onset of neuromuscular complications.

- Mental stress and tension which is a major factor in diabetes is controlled.

- There is a vast improvement in mood and behaviour of the individual.

- There is an increased sense of well being and optimistic approach to life.

- The immune system is boosted up which helps in combating various diseases in the body.

The Ragas Useful for Treatment of Diabetes

Research done in the medical application of Ragas have shown that the following Ragas are useful in the treatment of diabetes:

Raga Kalingara, Raga Hindol, Raga Bhairav, Raga Kafi, Raga Hansdhwani, Raga Bihag, Raga Malkauns, Raga Ramkali, Raga Bahar, Raga Deshkar, Raga Lalit, and Raga Jaijaiwanti.

Feng Shui

Feng Shui is the ancient Chinese art of living in harmony with the environment. It uses "Chi" (energy) to determine the positive and negative aspects of a home, office, building or factory environment.

Basic Philosophy

It is based on the theory that there is an invisible energy that flows through the universe, through our body, the food we eat, our home and work place and the environment around us. It is known as "prana" in India; "Chi" in China and "ki" in Japan.

According to a map or "Bagua" living spaces are divided into nine areas—career, knowledge, health, wealth, fame, relationships, children, travel and good luck. Energizing of these respective areas can enhance these qualities or areas of life.

	South			
	Wealth	Fame	Relationship	
East	Health	Good Luck	Children	West
	Knowledge	Career	Travel	
	North			

How it works?

It mainly works through colour schemes, placement of furniture, lighting, plants and reflective objects such as sculptures, paintings and art. To produce proper impact they should be so arranged that they are harmonious with the forces of nature or cosmic energy. Hence one can improve one's health, wealth, relationship, knowledge, career etc.

Feng Shui Measures for Treatment of Diabetes

The Health sector or the eastern portion of the house should be organized in such a way that all people including the diabetic individual live a long and healthy life. These measures are as follows:

- This room should be well-illuminated to allow increased amount of light which enables increased flow of "Chi" into this part of the house.

- Potted plants encourage good health and should form an integral part of the room.
- Photographs of family members and objects given by relatives, friends and well-wishers should be kept in the health sector.
- An aquarium or pictures depicting rivers, streams, waterfalls or lakes help in the well-being of occupants of the house.
- Keeping metallic wind chimes with hollow rods at the entrance or in the eastern portion help in the flow of beneficial "Chi" and remove all negative influences especially bad health.
- Keeping an orange or yenllow coloured bulb or candle lighted in this room during night is also useful.
- Painting the walls of the room with orange or yellow paint can keep all the occupants of the house fit and fine.
- There should be no clutter or useless things in this room which impede the free flow of energy into this room.
- The atmosphere can be further energized in this room by regular burning of incense or performing havan or "Kirtan" regularly.

8. What Does the Future Hold for Diabetes?

Diabetes mellitus is a modern-age epidemic estimated to affect about 150 million people in the world. India has the distinction of having 35 million diabetics in the country and has been declared by the World Health Organisation (WHO) as the Diabetes Capital of the World. WHO has estimated that the number of diabetic individuals in the world would reach 300 millions by the year 2025 and that of India 57 millions.

It is hoped that with the ongoing research on the causes, diagnosis and treatment of diabetes, the burden of diabetes would be definitely reduced in the near future.

Better Diagnostic Facilities
Revised Diagnostic Criteria
The newer diagnostic criteria proposed by the American Diabetes Association has brought out two new categories of diabetes - The impaired fasting glucose (IFG) and impaired glucose tolerance (IGT). Detection of these categories advocates prevention with lifestyle modification and diet to reverse them to normalcy. Some authors presume that these are pre-diabetic states.

Self-testing of Blood Sugar
Many electronic devices (glucometer/dextrometer) are available in the market using which the patient can find out his blood sugar values. Some devices have large digital displays or audio output to aid the visually impaired. Many portable, less expensive and sensitive instruments are available.

Continuous Glucose Monitors
Some companies have developed a blood glucose monitoring system which takes readings around the clock. An implantable monitor using a miniature sensor is also available. These monitors are very useful for patients on insulin therapy who need to know their blood sugar values regularly.

Glucose Watch
The gluco-watch biographer is a device like a wristwatch which provides blood glucose values every 20 minutes for 12 hours.

Better Treatment Modalities
Insulin Pens
Diabetic individuals who are on insulin can now use insulin pens which are self-contained injecting devices. There is no need to draw insulin into a syringe from a vial. The required dose can be dialled and injected using a plunger within it. Elderly people, blind, those with arthritis and children can benefit from these devices.

Painless Injections
Many drug companies have brought out injectable devices which are less painful than the traditional needle. Jet injectors eject insulin in a gaseous form which can penetrate the skin causing less pain and freedom from needle-phobia.

Nasal Insulin
Some companies have developed insulin which can be instilled into the nose and be absorbed into the bloodstream. It is painless, is quickly absorbed, but for a short period and produces nasal irritation.

Oral Spray
Oralin, a form of insulin that is sprayed into the mouth and absorbed through the cheek lining works well in controlling blood sugar in type-2 diabetes. In type-I diabetes it can be used in combination with insulin injections. It is absorbed more quickly, has no side-effects, is painless and will prove to be an effective alternative to insulin injections.

Insulin Pills

Insulin in the capsule form has so far not proved to be useful since it is destroyed by the digestive enzymes. Efforts are ongoing to make it safe from destruction by the digestive system.

Insulin Inhalers

Diabetes researchers have developed an inhaler-type of device which delivers fine aerosol droplets of insulin into the lungs as in the case of inhalers for asthma. These inhalers are also very useful for treatment of diabetes type-2.

Transdermal Patches

Insulin transdermal patches have been designed similar to nicotine patches used by smokers to give up smoking. These are patches worn on the skin and gradually absorbed into the bloodstreams. So far, results are disappointing.

Insulin Pumps

Certain insulin pumps have been devised which can be implanted under the skin or into the peritoneum. Using sensor mechanism they can detect as well as deliver insulin continuously. Miniature programmable pumps are very popular in the U.K. and U.S.A. among type-I diabetes patients.

Pancreas Transplant

Many scientists have tried transplantation of the whole or part of the pancreas from human cadaver (dead body) to diabetic individuals. Recently transplantation involves use of pancreatic islet cells which secrete insulin. To avoid rejection by the body, the transplanted cells are either surrounded by patient's own cells, or by barriers which prevent rejection. Some centres in the USA have developed techniques which involve hospitalization, only for 24-48 hours after minor surgery.

Newer Medicines

- Long-acting formulation of recently used medicines like glibenclamide, glipizide, gliclazide etc. will increase their absorption and enable early and sustained activity.

- A hormone from human intestine called Glucose-like-peptide-1 (GLP-1) helps in synchronizing insulin secretion with meal consumption. Injectable, inhaler and slow-releasing capsules of GLP-1 are under trial.

- Certain medicines have been developed which help in increasing secretion of insulin from the pancreas i.e. imidazoline compounds and phosphodiesterase inhibitors.

- Some newer medicines increase the activity of insulin like peroxisome-proliferator-activator-receptor-gamma (PPAR r), vanadium salts, insulin-like growth factor (IGF), lipoic acid, magnesium, chromium, vitamins C and E (antioxidants).

- Pramlintide injections help in diabetes control and also reduce body weight.

- Certain medicines help in preventing and delaying diabetic complications like protein-kinase C inhibitors, and angiogenic growth factor.

- The cost of insulin and other medicines have been reduced and their safety and efficacy enhanced.

- Special diabetic snacks and sweetening agents have been manufactured while diabetic individuals can enjoy without any increase in blood sugar levels.

Gene therapy

Insulin gene therapy involves introducing a foreign gene into any type of cell in the human body to allow it to produce insulin. Islet cells are derived from human embryo (baby) or adult or animal pancreas.

The latest technique is transdifferentiation in which a gene is inserted into patient's liver cells converting them into islet cells. These cells once converted into islet cells cannot revert back. Thus a part of the liver can be converted into the pancreas and rest of it can carry on its normal liver functions.

Gene therapy will definitely help in "curing" diabetes in the years to come.

■■■

9. Answers to Your Queries

1. What is diabetes and how is it caused?

   Diabetes is a disease in which the body is unable to metabolize the carbohydrates in the diet and provide glucose to all parts of the body. It is due to lack of production of a hormone called insulin in the pancreas or due to inefficient action of insulin.

2. How many varieties of diabetes do occur?

   The two major varieties of diabetes are type-1 and type-2 diabetes. Type-1 diabetes is controlled only by insulin injections and type-2 diabetes by oral medicines.

3. Can it occur in children?

   Yes, type-1 diabetes is usually common in children and can occur from infancy to adolescence.

4. Is there any specific age-group where diabetes occur?

   No, diabetes can affect any age-group.

5. Is it true that is can occur only in obese individuals?

   Not necessarily. Type-2 diabetes usually occurs in obese individuals, but type-1 can occur in individuals who are normal or underweight.

6. Does it occur in people who consume a lot of sweets?

   Usually not, but if weight is gained it may aggravate the underlying tendency towards the disease.

7. Is diabetes inherited?

   Yes, if both parents have diabetes, the probability is that some of their children will develop the disease in their lifetime.

8. Does stress affect diabetes?

   Yes, physical and mental stress can unmask diabetes or aggravate it.

9. Is it more common in urban or rural areas and why?

   Recent research has shown that it is more common in urban areas due to sedentary lifestyle, high-caloric diet and stress.

10. Does our lifestyle have any bearing on the disease?

    Definitely. High-caloric diet, lack of exercise, smoking, alcoholism, and stressful occupation can give rise to diabetes in prone individuals and also produce poor control of the disease.

11. Is diabetes a contagious disease?

    Never. By mere contact or living with a person suffering from diabetes, one cannot acquire this disease.

12. Is it common during pregnancy?

    Yes, diabetes can occur during pregnancy and can produce complications both in the mother and baby.

13. Can certain medicines cause or aggravate diabetes?

    Yes, certain medicines like oral diuretics (used to increase passage of urine), adrenaline, oral pills, corticosteroids, rat poison (valcor), cassava and certain beans can cause or aggravate diabetes.

14. Are there any specific symptoms which warn us about the disease?

    There are no specific symptoms which definitely point out towards diabetes. Symptoms like increased thirst and appetite, loss of weight inspite of good food intake, frequent injections, unexplained weakness and impotence may be seen as warning symptoms in some individuals.

15. For diagnosis of diabetes, which test is more relevant–urine or blood sugar?

    Blood sugar testing is more accurate than urine sugar testing. Urine sugar is present usually when the blood sugar levels are very high (about 180mg%).

16. Can we test diabetes at home too?

    Yes. Certain portable devices (glucometer) can help in estimating blood sugar levels at home.

17. What is HbA_{1c} test?

    This is a blood test used to determine the blood sugar control in the last three months. It is very useful in type-1 diabetes where there are wide fluctuations in blood sugar levels.

18. What are the organs which can be damaged if diabetes is present for a long time?

    Diabetes of long duration can damage the heart, kidney, eyes, nerves and feet.

19. Can low blood sugar ever occur in diabetic individuals?

    Yes. Those who take medicines/injections without proper meals or in improper doses, with alcohol or after an excessive exercise, can develop low blood sugar (hypoglycemia).

20. What is keto-acidosis?

    Keto-acidosis is a major emergency which can occur due to untreated or uncontrolled diabetes.

21. What is the role of diet in diabetic control?

    In type-2 diabetes, intake of calories should be reduced to reduce weight. Moreover, loss of carbohydrates and fats play a positive role in diabetic control except in malnourished individuals.

22. Can regular exercise help in diabetic control?

    Yes. Regular exercise helps in controlling diabetes by weight reduction, increased efficiency of insulin and control of blood pressure and kidney functions.

23. Can a diabetic individual increase the dose of his medicine/ injection when he eats more than his allowance?

    Not without the consent of the treating doctor, as it can upset the control of the disease.

24. Can diabetic individuals keep a fast?

    Type-2 obese diabetics may benefit by keeping a fast but type-1 diabetics who are under weight and on large doses of insulin should avoid it or reduce the dose of insulin.

25. Can a diabetic individual use medicines for reducing weight?

    Preferably not, since most medicines are appetite suppressants which stimulate the nervous system and have minimal effect on weight control. The long-term effects of herbal medicines are not known and hence should be avoided.

26. Is it true that once insulin is started, it has to be taken life-long and also oral medicines will not be effective?

    This is partially true. Type-1 diabetes individuals have no endogenous insulin and have to depend on insulin for life. Type-2 diabetes individuals usually have their diabetes controlled with oral medicines. They may require insulin during infections, surgery, stress or when diabetes is not adequately controlled. Insulin is usually discontinued once the diabetes is brought under control and patient continues on oral medicines.

27. If an overdose of insulin is given unknowingly, what will happen and how can it be controlled?

    Usually it leads to hypoglycemia or low blood sugar symptoms like hunger pains, sweating, feeling of weakness, numbness of lips and fingers, pounding heart, headache, drowsiness, confusion may occur. A cube of sugar or 10-20gm of glucose powder may be given and the doctor informed.

28. Why are cramps in the legs more common in individuals with diabetes?

    Cramps in the legs are due to damage to the nerves which is common in diabetic individuals, especially of type-2 variety.

29. Is diabetes curable?

    Diabetes cannot be cured, but can be controlled by diet regulation, regular exercise and medicines/insulin injections.

30. If one forgets to take insulin in the morning, can he take a double dose in the evening?

    No. This might lead to hypoglycemia.

31. Is it true that heart attack is painless in diabetics?

    Yes. Mostly heart attack is painless or silent. It can be diagnosed with the help of an ECG. Warning signs are breathlessness and choking sensation.

32. Can we find out whether the kidneys have been affected by diabetes and how?

    Yes. We can find out by the presence of a protein called albumin in the urine. In advanced kidney disease, blood urea or creatmine will be increased.

33. Can sexual activity be affected in a diabetic individual?

    Yes. Uncontrolled diabetes can lead to impotence. There is an urge but it is often difficult to perform. This problem occurs in long-standing uncontrolled diabetes.

34. Can a diabetic be safely operated upon?

    Yes. In such cases, usually insulin is used to control blood sugar levels before, during and after the surgery or operation.

35. Are menstruation and menopause affected by diabetes?

    Young diabetic females are known to start their periods slightly later than normal girls and have irregular cycles. Menopause is difficult to diagnose due to repeated episodes of low blood sugar which resemble hot flushes.

36. Can diabetic people seek any kind of job?

    Type-1 diabetics who are on insulin treatment and frequently develop low blood sugar levels or ketosis are unfit for the following jobs:

    Jobs with irregular working hours or shifts, frequent touring or driving, heavy manual work, working at heights, working with or near a heavy moving or high-voltage machinery, working alone, especially at night, working in armed forces, police or fire department. Risky jobs like diving, mining, aircraft driving, mountaineering etc. should also be avoided.

37. Is long distance travel prohibited for diabetics?

    No, but certain precautions should be taken regarding diet and medicines, especially in those with type-1 diabetes. If you are driving you may need extra calories than usual and also while walking long distances or climbing mountains.

38. Does alcohol intake affect diabetic individuals?

    Yes, especially on an empty stomach. Alcohol can produce hypoglycemia alone as well as after reacting with the anti-diabetic medications. Since the symptoms of excessive alcohol as well as hypoglycemia are similar, the latter may not be detected and can be fatal at times.

39. Can all diabetics take part in sports/exercise?

    Yes, but should adjust doses of their medicine and diet to avoid episodes of hypoglycemia which is very common.

40. Can all medicines be used along with anti-diabetic medications/insulin?

    No. Certain medicines, especially those used for hypertension, cough syrups, diuretics, steroids, hormones, painkillers etc. should be used with caution since they may increase or decrease blood sugar levels.

41. Can a diabetic lady safely breastfeed her newborn baby?

    No, many of the medicines (oral) used to control diabetes enter the mother's milk and may be passed on to the baby. So in majority of cases, insulin is the best form of treatment.

42. Are diabetic individuals more prone to infections than non-diabetic individuals?

    Yes, to a large extent, since their immune-system is weak and high blood sugar levels enhance the growth of bacteria, viruses and other micro-organisms. Hence, they also require a prolonged course of antibiotics and other medicines for treatment.

43. Is it true that diabetic individuals are prone to have an amputation of their feet or legs?

    Yes. Due to improper blood circulation and nerve supply, blood vessels in the legs and feet have a tendency to undergo degenerative changes and eventually gangrene. This can often lead to amputation of the leg or foot to save the remaining part of the limb.

44. Can eyes be affected in diabetes?

    Yes. In chronic diabetes the eyes are affected and give rise to cataract, glaucoma, myopia (shortsightedness) and even blindness due to involvement of retina.

45. Can excessive smoking affect diabetic control?

    Yes. Nicotine from cigarettes can increase insulin requirements and also increase complications in the blood vessels affecting the heart, kidneys, eyes and feet.

46. Are there any recent changes in the values of blood sugar suggestive of diabetes?

    Yes. The American Diabetes Association has recommended that the fasting blood sugar values of more than 126mg% and post-prandial (after 2 hours) more than 200mg% are diagnostic of diabetes. The fasting values of 110-125mg% and post-prandial values of 140-199mg% are suggestive of intermediate stage of the disease.

47. How frequently should blood sugar tests be done?

    Patients with type-1 diabetes should get their blood sugar test done daily while those with type-2 diabetes once weekly till normal values are attained.

48. What is the role of sweeteners in diabetes?

    Sweeteners like aspartame (Equal, Sugar-free, Sweetex, Aspasweet etc) contain sucrose which can be safely used in diabetics to enhance the taste of their food without increasing caloric intake.

49. Do yoga and alternative therapies have a role in controlling diabetes?

    Yes. Recent research has shown that yoga and other alternative therapies can control diabetes and even reduce the doses of insulin and oral medicines. But their curative value is not known.

50. What is magnitude of incidence of diabetes in India?

    India is known as the Diabetes Capital of the world. Out of 150 million diabetic people in the world, India is estimated to have about 35 million diabetics at present (Novo Nordisk).

■■■

10. Role of Commonly Available Ayurvedic Medicines

Due to the rapid increase in the incidence and complications of Diabetes Mellitus in India, many pharmaceutical companies have started to explore the nature's flora for an answer. This has resulted in the manufacturing boom of several ayurvedic (herbomineral) preparations in the market. The pharmaceutical companies are in the process of striking a goldmine both in Indian and overseas markets by claiming that these medicines are curative, free from any side-effects and give permanent relief from diabetes.

A critical analysis of these ayurvedic medicines is given below. The table below shows the important herbomineral medicines available in the market and their important ingredients.

Name of the Medicine	Pharmaceutical Company	Important Ingredients
Diabecon	Himalaya Drug Co.	Meshashringi, Pitasara, Saptarangi, Jambu, Guduchi, Shilajit, Guggulu, Punarnava, Kairata, Bhumyamalaki
Hyponidd	Charaka Pharmaceuticals	Jambu, Gudmar, Pitasara, Shilajit, Haridra, Kairata, Trivanga Bhasma, Guduchi
Glucomap	Maharishi Ayurvedics	Jambu, Nimba, Arjuna, Shilajit, Nagajihwa, Bhumyamalaki, Bilva, Salasaradigana, Karavellaka

Name of the Medicine	Pharmaceutical Company	Important Ingredients
X-Diaba	Surya Herbal	Gudmar, Karela beeja, Jamun seed, Neem, Methi, Shilajit, Kasani, Basanta Kusumakara Rasa, Trivanga Bhasma, Vijaysara, Giloy
Madhumehari	Baidyanath	Gudmar, Haridra, Amalaki, Kairata, Udumbura Phala, Methi seeds, Bijaka, Jamun seeds, Khadira, Amritha, Nimba, Bilva
Amree Plus	Aimil Pharmaceuticals	Gudmar, Karela, Vijaysara, Bilva, Jamun, Tejpatra, Shilajit, Methi, Kalmegh, Chandra Prabha Vati, Neem, Giloe, Swaran Makshik Bhasam, Sadabahar, Bhringraj, Punarnava, Bimbi, Aloe vera (Kumari/Kunwar Patha), Sharpunkha
Gludibit	Lupin Herbals	Madhunashini, Vijaysara, Mamumajjak, Nimba, Saptachakra
Cogent-db+	Cybele Herbal Laboratories Pvt. Ltd.	Neem, Methi, Haridra, Trifla, Jamun, Gokshura
Glucorid-kp	Dabur Ayurvedic Specialities	Karela freeze dried powder, Gudmar
Jambrulin	Unjha Pharma Pvt. Ltd. Works Ltd.	Jamun seeds, Mammajjak, Bilva, Trivanga Bhasma, Gudmar, Neem, Shilajit
Tribangshila	Zandu Pharmaceuticals	Trivanga Bhasma, Neem, Gudmar, Mammajjak, Jamun, Bitumen.

A critical analysis of medicines available in the market has shown that majority of the medicines have ingredients to serve the following purposes:

- Stimulate the secretion of insulin from the pancreas, which is the major defect in Diabetes.
- Improve the carbohydrate metabolism and thereby reduce the glucose (sugar) levels in the blood.

- Enhance the fat metabolism to reduce the level of cholesterol, lipids & triglycerides which can also help in preventing complications of heart & brain (stroke) & ketosis.
- Symptomatic relief of symptoms like increased thirst, urination, tiredness etc.
- Certain ingredients are capable of preventing complications of kidneys (albuminuria), eye (retinopathy), infections of skin and genitourinary system.
- Some ayurvedic ingredients can reduce increased body weight, which is the basic cause of type 2 diabetes.
- Some medicines have the capacity to boost immune system of the body, which is very important in combating various infections and complications of diabetes.
- Some formulations improve therapeutic response to conventional allopathic medicines, reduce dependence on them and even reduce their doses and side effects.

Mechanism of Action of Common Ingredients

1. **Gudmar,** also known as **Meshashringi** & **Madhunashini** is a woody climber whose leaves have a medicinal value, containing gymnemic acid, which increases secretion of insulin by pancreas and enhances utilization of glucose by tissues. Gudmar is also capable of repairing and regenerating weak damaged beta cells of pancreas, which produce insulin.

2. **Vijayasar** or **Pitasara** or **Bijaka** is a large deciduous tree whose bark has a medicinal value. The bark contains certain compounds, which have insulin-like properties. It decreases blood sugar levels by increasing utilization of glucose by the tissues & by reducing glucose absorption from intestines. It can also increase insulin levels in pancreas & regenerate beta cells.

3. **Jambu** or **Jamun** tree is an evergreen tree, whose seeds contain jamboline, which is useful in patients with Diabetes. Jamboline prevents conversion of starch into sugar & also diminishes quantity of sugar in urine & reduces thirst.

4. **Karavella** or **Sushavi**, commonly known as **Karela**, is a climber cultivated as a vegetable crop. The fruit contains certain insulin-like compounds, which reduce blood glucose levels & also help in stimulating release of insulin from pancreas. It can also decrease elevated blood cholesterol levels & also prevent ketosis.

5. **Shilajit** or Mineral Pitch is known to relieve thirst, increased urination & exhaustion & helps in assimilation of sugar. It acts as a biocatalyst, increases peripheral demand of glucose, & has an anabolic action. It prevents deterioration of pancreatic cells by restricting glucose load & promoting unrestricted insulin activity. It is useful in diabetic albuminuria (kidney disorder).

6. **Guduchi** is known to reduce blood sugar levels significantly. It also promotes insulin-induced glucose uptake by tissues. It increases the immunity of the body and enhances the sense of well-being.

7. **Punarnava** is an abundantly grown herb, whose root contains an alkaloid-punarnavine. This alkaloid has property of protecting heart by reducing the levels of lipids (fats) in the blood, thus preventing heart attack & stroke. It increases urination, thereby protecting kidneys from disease.

8. **Guggulu** is the gum-resin which exudes from the bark of a small shrub found in dry, rocky areas. It has capacity to reduce cholesterol & other fats in blood and thus prevent cardiac complications of diabetes. It also helps in decreasing body weight in obese, which is very essential for patients with type 2 diabetes.

9. **Trifla** contains Harad, Baheda & Amla which have the rejuvenating and anti-aging properties. Trifla helps in maintaining normal function of blood vessels, nerves and eyes (retina) and prevents diabetic complications in these tissues.

10. **Neem leaves** have antiseptic properties and are useful in healing diabetic foot, gangrene & acts as a blood purifier & protects blood vessels against disease.

11. **Haridra (Haldi)** is known for its antiseptic properties since time immemorial. It is a powerful blood purifier & helps in healing chronic wounds including gangrene of diabetic foot.

12. **Gokshura** is a medicinal plant useful in problems of urinary system. It prevents damage to kidney, improves kidney function & prevents impotence, which is very common in diabetes.

13. **Saptarangi or Saptachakra** is another medicinal plant whose bark contains certain compounds, which promote insulin induced glucose uptake by tissues & reduces blood sugar levels.

14. **Bhumyamalaki** leaves have capacity to reduce blood sugar very effectively.

15. **Abhraka Bhasma** is prepared from biotite, processed with juices & extracts of various plants that makes it a potent cellular regenerator. It is very useful in controlling diabetes & urinary infections.

16. **Pravala Bhasma** contains calcium, magnesium, iron & their compounds which help in treating carbuncles & other skin infections associated with diabetes.

17. **Vanga Bhasma** is prepared from tin & is found to be very effective in treatment of infections of genitourinary system.

18. Other important herbal ingredients are extracts of methi seeds, tulsi leaves, tej patta, Kumari (Kanwar Patha), Kutaki, Kalmegh, Gular, Mammajjak (Nagjivha or Nahhi), Yastimadhu, Bhringraj, Shatavari, Mundatika, Karpasi, Bilva, Rohitaka, Maricha, Vishnupriya, Atibala, Kairatikta, Jungli Palak, Bimbi, Sadabahar, Vidangi Loham, Swaran Makshik Bhasma, Yashad Bhasma.

It may be concluded that different Ayurvedic pharmaceutical companies have different ingredients in their products, each having property of reducing blood sugar levels. However, so far no product is available having curative properties. These medicines may be used as an adjuvant therapy alongwith other allopathic medicines. They may have an additive effect alongwith conventional medicines & in some cases the doses & adverse effects of Allopathic medicines may be reduced.

www.ingramcontent.com/pod-product-compliance
Lightning Source LLC
Chambersburg PA
CBHW070335230426
43663CB00011B/2320